COLOUR ME BEAUTIFUL

COLOUR ME BEAUTIFUL

DISCOVER YOUR NATURAL BEAUTY THROUGH COLOUR

CAROLE JACKSON

PIATKUS

Also by Carole Jackson
Colour Me Beautiful Make-Up Book

All models appearing in *Colour Me Beautiful* were photographed by David Neely, Photo Concepts.

A special thanks to
Dorothy Douse and Frances Roller for appearing in
Colour Me Beautiful

All other models in *Colour Me Beautiful* are from
The Model Store, Washington, D.C.

Katie Brown	Jennifer Klouman
Trena Brown	Terri Moller
Margaret Connelly	Holly O'Dell
Barbara Evans	Lisa Sanders
Betsy Farley	Kim Shanahan
Colleen Gaschen	Maura Shea
Mary Heron	Laurie Solow
Pam Harris	Susan Volk

Make-up and Hair Styling by Susan Volk

© 1980 Acropolis Books Ltd, Washington D.C.

First published in Great Britain in 1983 by
Judy Piatkus (Publishers) Ltd of
5 Windmill Street, London W1

Reprinted 1983, 1985, 1986 (twice),
1988, 1989 (twice), 1990, 1991,
1992, 1993, 1994, 1995

UK *Colour Me Beautiful* consultant Madge Campbell
UK edition designed by Alan Coombes

ISBN 0 86188 299 7

Printed and bound in Great Britain by
The Bath Press, Bath, Avon

CONTENTS

ACKNOWLEDGEMENTS

This book has been fun to write. Everyone became involved, because colour is contagious. People all along the chain of creating and promoting *Colour Me Beautiful* are now wearing their colours.

To those who gave their time and talent beyond the call of friendship or a pay cheque, I give special thanks. First of all, to my associates in colour, Mary Murphy and Sari Martin, who teach our classes in Scarsdale, New York. And then, for reasons they each know best, Winifred A. Adams, Cozy Baker, Bill B., Jeanne Brodsky, Andy Cella, Suzanne Greene, Kathleen Hughes, Margot Kline, Barbara Moore, Tom and Carla Nankervis, and Sandy Stewart. And especially, to John, for his thoughtful input, sensitivity, and friendship, and to Alec and Megan, for their enthusiasm and helpfulness from start to finish.

It is with equal gratitude that I acknowledge the women (and men) who have taken my classes and shared with me the joy of finding their colours.

INTRODUCTION

THE MAGIC OF COLOUR

When I was a young girl, I wanted so much to be pretty. Studying myself in the mirror, I saw a pale, colourless face and decided that I really wasn't pretty at all. While the powder blue uniform required at my school made some of the girls look marvellous it did nothing for me. It in fact made me look grey, dull, and lifeless. The colour of that daily uniform robbed me of some potentially good feelings about myself well into adult life.

Discovering lipstick and rouge as a teenager brought me instant life, but it was not until years later that I discovered the real magic of colour. MY colours . . . the missing link to finding my best self.

After having my colouring analysed by a professional colour consultant, I found that I do not look pale and lifeless after all – as long as I wear a colour (the right blue, for example) that brings out the glow of my natural colouring. As I began wearing only the colours that were right for me, I started receiving compliments *all the time*. My colours had such an impact on my life that I wanted to share this exciting concept with others. You have special colours, too.

Each of us has a unique skin tone. Finding the colours that best complement this tone brings out our special beauty. I have seen many women literally come to life with radiance and new-found self-confidence as they discover their colours.

Perhaps you have never thought much about colour, but I promise you that colour has more impact than you ever imagined! Artists have studied its secrets and use them to make their masterpieces come alive. The world's most beautiful women – and men – have discovered its power to make the world regard them with awe.

Why do you picture Elizabeth Taylor in vivid, clear colours – royal blue, emerald green – and Candice Bergen in pastels? Why did your friend look fabulous on Monday, yet why did you walk right past her on Tuesday without saying hello because you didn't notice her? Why do you always reach for that certain dress in your own wardrobe? The answer is *colour*.

Nine years ago, after formal study of colour and its application to clothing, makeup, and hair, I set up classes to teach women of all ages how to put themselves together from head to toe using their colours as the foundation. Over the years these classes have been refined, and they are the basis for this book.

At these 'Colour Me Beautiful' classes, we analyse each client's colouring, give her a packet of fabric swatches in her colour palette, and teach her how to use them as a guide for shopping and looking beautiful. We also cover makeup and hair, clothing personality and style, and wardrobe planning.

We use the seasons to describe people's colouring. For just as nature has divided herself into four distinct seasons, Autumn, Spring, Winter, and Summer, each with its unique and harmonious colours, your genes have given you a type of colouring that is most complemented by one of these seasonal palettes.

An Autumn person radiates in the warm, rich autumnal colours, with their golden undertones, as crisp and colourful as the October leaves. A Spring blossoms in clear, delicate colours with warm yellow undertones, like the first daffodil that blooms each spring. A Winter sparkles in the vivid, clear primary colours, and cool, icy colours, like a glittering snowflake. And a Summer person glows in the pastels of June, the soft colours of the sea and sky, with their cool, blue undertones.

Through this book you will discover *your* season and learn which colours make you look fabulous all the time. After you know your best colours, you will move on to learn exactly what makeup and hair tones are perfect for you. Then we'll plan your wardrobe.

Colour *is* magic and now let it work for you!

PART ONE

FIND YOUR COLOURS, FIND YOURSELF

CHAPTER ONE

LET'S START WITH YOU

The first step in finding the colours that are perfect for you is a self-evaluation. Your answers to the following questions may help you increase your awareness of your clothes-buying and beauty habits. In addition, believe it or not, each question relates to colour.

1. Can you wear *any* colour and look your best?

2. Do you create a good first impression *all the time*?

3. Do you have a wardrobe full of clothes but nothing to wear?

4. Do you feel guilty about spending money on clothes?

5. Are you a compulsive clothes buyer?

6. Are there any mistakes hanging in your wardrobe?

7. When you shop, do you have direction, or do you wander aimlessly? Are you sure that everything you buy will be just right for you and will blend with the rest of your wardrobe?

8. Can you pack one suitcase for a two-week trip?

9. Do you buy too much makeup, or no makeup at all, because you aren't sure what is just right for you?

10. If you colour your hair, are you positive that it is the most flattering shade?

11. Are you excited about the way you look?

12. Do you have 'colourisma'?

If any *one* of your answers does not please you, *Colour Me Beautiful* can help. By finding and learning to use your special colours, you can achieve just what you want, whether it's a little change here and there, or an entirely new look. Then you can be happy with your answers to all these questions, for colour – your personal palette – makes all the pieces fall into place. You'll look better; you'll shop more intelligently; and – if you're like the women who have taken my classes – you'll be excited about your looks and yourself.

CHAPTER TWO

COLOUR MAKES THE DIFFERENCE

Everyone is born with an inclination towards certain colours. I have found that a very young child, before being influenced by parents and peers, will invariably pick out colours that suit her, sometimes to the horror of mother. One of my clients brought in her four-year-old for a colour analysis. 'Every time we go shopping she wants a black dress!' wailed the frustrated parent. The child was a Winter and black was indeed her colour. Mother was a Spring, at home in camel and peach.

By the time we grow up, we may have lost a portion of that personal colour sense, and we buy colours for reasons that don't have anything to do with how we look in them. We have been bombarded with colour messages from mother (whose best colours may be different from our own) and from the fashion and home-furnishings industries.

Take heart. Nature usually prevails, and chances are good that at least 50 percent of your clothes are the right colours. And you probably already know which ones they are; they're the ones that make you feel attractive and confident. Soon all your clothes will make you feel that way.

I was a bit sceptical when I had my colours analysed years ago, but when I tried one of my new shades, the result was remarkable. I chose a royal blue turtleneck, a daring colour for me, and wore it to a meeting one night when my mood was down. As I walked through the door, I received a compliment (a compliment to *me*, not my sweater). Dubious of this unexpected praise, I glanced in the mirror and discovered that I did indeed look better than I felt. My mood changed. By the end of the evening, after many compliments, I felt radiant. I knew my colours were working for me.

Let me tell you about a few of the people who have enjoyed the very positive benefits of colour analysis.

Jenny came to me in the middle of her diet. She had lost four stones, had four more to go, and there was no stopping her. She was thrilled with her colours and had the pleasure of replacing her wardrobe quickly because she was rapidly growing too small for her clothes. Fortunately, she was developing self esteem and was willing to buy attractive clothes even though she planned to be too small for them the next year (she was). My phone rang for months as Jenny's friends saw her transformation and wanted the same for themselves.

Pam was depressed. She had lost the ability to make even minor decisions and really had lost interest in life. A friend dragged her to my classes in hopes of cheering her up. She was obviously pleased with the reactions of the class as we draped her in her colours. But she was still afraid to go shopping. I finally gave her an assignment. She was to go to a department store and buy one blouse (which she said she needed). The next week, she came in beaming. 'It was so easy,' she said. 'I didn't even look at half the things on the rack because they weren't my colours. I only took a few blouses into the dressing room and the second one I tried on looked so good that I didn't bother with the others. I bought it and here I am.'

Marnie was a Summer whose hair had darkened. Her mother was an Autumn, and Marnie had spent her childhood in Autumn colours. Even now she wore mostly earth colours. She felt drab and wanted to do something to her hair, but she wasn't sure what. Draping her in Summer colours brought her to life. She was radiant. She highlighted her hair just the right shade and looked stunning. Marnie also sells cosmetics and has found that her understanding of the seasonal palettes helps her tremendously with her clients.

'Help!' said Kathy. 'I need a new image.' Kathy was overweight and came to class in blue jeans, with her blonde hair in two bunches. At thirty-three, she obviously hadn't found herself. By the end of the six-week course, she had shed a stone, sported a chic, short haircut, and looked fabulous in her new makeup and a skirt and blouse in her colours. Six weeks later she had lost another stone and had found a whole new identity. Kathy was one of my first students, and six years later, I am happy to report that she is still skinny, and looks great.

Helen came to me right after her divorce. She had gone back to college, at fifty, to prepare herself for re-entry into the job market. Her colours, makeup, and a wardrobe plan for a working woman brought her up-to-date. She later wrote: 'Getting my colours is the nicest thing I've done for myself in years. I felt so good during my job interviews, and I am sure my new boss thinks I'm ten years younger than I am!'

Marie was laughing when she came to the last class. 'I went to my doctor and he wouldn't believe I wasn't feeling well because I look so good.' Marie was a pale Autumn who had never worn makeup. To camouflage the grey that was creeping into her hair, she had tinted it a silvery ash blonde – wrong for her. With her colours, a little rouge and lipstick, and a change to auburn hair, she was indeed a new woman.

The discovery of colour transformed each of these women. Colour does make a difference – often a dramatic one. The fun is in the discovery; the rewards last a lifetime.

WRONG COLOUR   **RIGHT COLOUR**

Margaret

Margaret is a Winter with grey-blue eyes, dark ash brown hair and fair skin with a blue undertone. Her colouring is best complemented by clothes and makeup in cool, clear colours. In the picture on the left she is wearing a gold shirt and orange-toned makeup. She looks pale and plain. But in the picture on the right, she is wearing royal blue with cool-toned makeup: a blue-red lipstick and pink rouge. See how radiant she looks!

SUMMER   AUTUMN

Mary   *Kim*

Mary and Kim both have green eyes and brown hair, yet they are different seasons. Mary has a pink skin tone and looks best in cool colours with blue undertones, like the fuchsia she is wearing above. Kim's skin is ivory with golden highlights and she is most flattered by warm colours with yellow undertones, as in her orange sweater. Mary is a Summer; Kim is an Autumn. Notice that Mary's hair has a taupe (greyish) cast while Kim's hair has golden red highlights. Mary's green eyes have a hint of blue in them; Kim's green eyes, however, have gold tones.

Many green- or brown-eyed Summers mistakenly think they are Autumns. In the pictures on the right Mary and Kim are wearing the same two turtlenecks, camel from the Autumn palette and pink from the Summer palette. Each changed her lipstick and blusher to go with the colour of her shirt. See how Summer Mary looks drab in the yellow-tone camel and orange lipstick, but comes to life in the pink shirt and pink makeup tones that are so complementary to her natural colouring. By contrast, Kim is pale in the cool pink tones, but looks bright and healthy in the camel shirt and orange-tone makeup.

WRONG COLOUR   **RIGHT COLOUR**

WRONG COLOUR

RIGHT COLOUR

Susan

Susan, a Spring, has an ivory skin tone, clear green eyes, and golden blonde hair. She looks best when she wears clear, yellow-toned colours. On the left she is wearing pure white, which drains the colour from her face. But when she wears the coral pink sweater, in the picture on the right, her face comes to life – even in the same makeup. Susan's best white is ivory, a creamy white with a yellow undertone. Place a piece of ivory paper over her white sweater and see how much more flattering the ivory is. A Winter is the only season who is truly flattered by pure white.

CHAPTER THREE

THE SEASONAL PALETTES

Mirror, mirror, on the wall, who's the fairest of them all? You are!

Nature is the most brilliant designer of all, and the secret is in her seasons. Each season presents a distinct array of colours, and *your* colouring is in harmony with one of these palettes. We could call your colouring 'Type A,' 'Type B,' and so on, but comparison with the seasons provides a more aesthetic and poetic way to describe your colouring and your best colours.

Some women are their most beautiful in the clear, true primary colours or the icy colours of Winter, while others are flattered more by the softer shades of Summer. Autumns come to life in rich, warm tones, and the Spring woman's colouring is most enhanced by clear, warm colours, like the budding growth and fresh fruit tones of springtime. When you wear your special colours, you are indeed the fairest of them all.

The genes that determine your skin tone, hair, and eye colour also determine what colours look best on you. When you study your colouring, you will find that your skin, hair, and eyes have either blue or golden tones. Your inherited skin tone does not change; it simply deepens with a tan and fades with age. The same colours – whether they are the cool colours of Winter and Summer, or the warm tones of Autumn and Spring – will always look the best on you.

In our classes, we drape each client in all the colours of her season, contrasting wrong colours for the sake of comparison and illustration. The right colour brings out the best, while the wrong shade detracts. It's exciting to see the differences. Many women do not know how pretty they are.

You can then go on to match your makeup to your colours, and learn which hair tones are right for you.

First you must examine the seasonal palettes on pages 27 to 33.

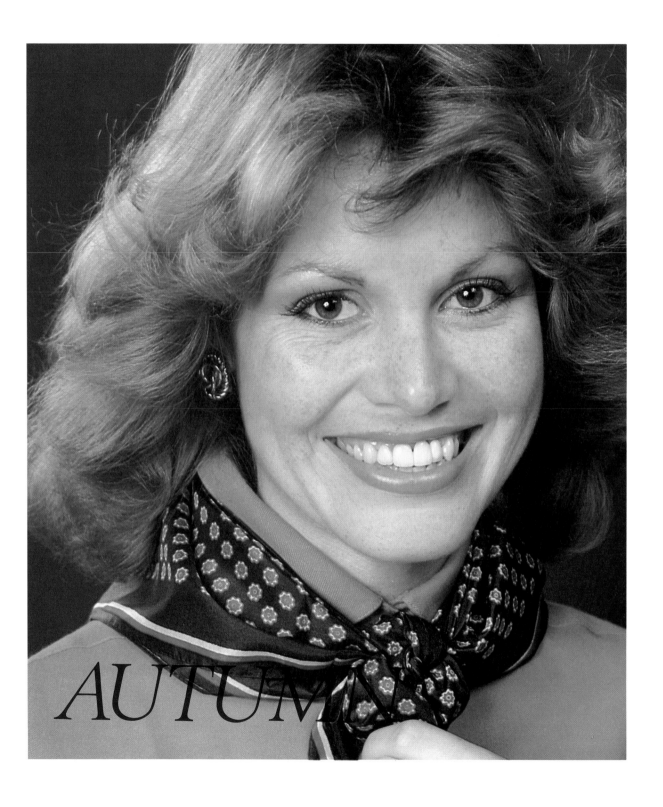

THE PALETTES

Before you take the colour test, let's look carefully at the palettes on pages 27 to 33. The Winter palette has either blue-based colours or true colours – colours with a balance between yellow and blue, black and white. The Summer colours have either blue, rose, or grey undertones. Because of these undertones, Winter and Summer are the *cool* palettes. Autumn's colours are based on golden tones, and Spring's have clear, yellow undertones. These are the *warm* palettes. Your colouring, like your palette, is either cool (blue) or warm (golden).

Study the characteristics of each seasonal palette, noting especially the differences in the beiges, blues, greens, pinks, and reds. Do you see, for example, that the Spring palette has clear yellow-greens, while Autumn has both yellow-greens and earth greens? Winter's greens are true or icy, and the Summer palette contains only blue-greens. Summers and Winters wear blue-reds (cool), while Springs and Autumns look best in orange-reds (warm). Spring's pinks have yellow in them; Summer's are blue-pinks; Winter's are true and vivid or icy; and Autumn has no pink.

Now examine the palettes for intensity. Although Winter and Summer are both cool, the depth of their colours varies considerably. The same is true of Autumn's and Spring's warm palettes. Winter's colours are all clear, true, vivid, or icy, while Summer's colours may be either clear or powdered (muted) and are always less intense. While Winter has royal purple, Summer has plum, a muted purple. Note the differences in the intensity of the blues, pinks, greens, and yellows. Note, too, the differences in the Winter and Summer models. Winter colouring is stronger, with greater contrast in skin, hair, and eyes. Summer has softer, less intense colouring. The warm Autumn palette is strong, with both vivid and muted colours. But Spring has only *clear* colours, either bright or delicate, but never muted or extremely dark. Notice the differences in the golds, browns, greens, beiges, and oranges of these two seasons. See how much darker the Autumn models' hair and eyes are compared to the delicate colouring of the Spring models.

A few colours are missing entirely from some of the palettes, and other colours are unique to just one palette. Winter is the only season to have black and pure white. But Winter has no brown or orange. Autumn alone has very dark brown, but no navy, pink, or grey. Summer has no orange, and Spring has a little bit of every colour except black and pure white.

In looking at the palettes, you may feel that you can wear colours from all the seasons. True, it is possible to find a few colours from each that might suit you. Some colours are relatively flattering to everyone, which is nice if you need to dress a bevy of bridesmaids. Everyone can wear

Summer's soft white (this is not a yellow-white). Other good colours for a group are Spring's corals and her light warm aqua, Autumn's deep periwinkle blue, and Summer's watermelon. These colours are not included in all the palettes, however, because they are a compromise for some.

There are two important reasons for *not* mixing palettes or 'borrowing' colours from a palette that is not yours. First, you will look *best* in your own colours. Second, each palette has been carefully arranged to give you a well-coordinated wardrobe, consisting of compatible tones. If you buy colours at random, you will end up with loads of clothes and nothing to wear. As you build your wardrobe from the palette of your season, you will quickly benefit from this bonus. Because your colours go with each other, your outfits and accessories will coordinate all by themselves. Perhaps you fear being restricted or bored wearing only one set of colours. But look at the variety in each season! Once into your palette, you will find instead that you have more colours to wear than you currently allow yourself – perhaps colours you never thought of trying. The truth is that you can wear almost any *colour;* it's the *shade and intensity* that count! We are going to enrich and enlarge your wardrobe possibilities to some thirty shades that all look good on you. You won't be bored by your colours, and it's never boring to be beautiful.

The palettes are all designed to give you a wide range of colours, with something appropriate for every time of year and for every kind of occasion. Some of your colours are suitable for wintertime, some for summertime. Your palette contains sporty colours, dressy colours, neutrals, basics, and bright accent colours. You will find a colour to suit your every mood and need.

The seasonal colour theory was inspired by the studies of artist and colourist Johannes Itten of the famous Bauhaus school in Germany. He discovered the power of physical colouring in directing a student's choice of colours in his paintings. He noted that a student's personal colours were consistently those complementary to his skin tone, hair, and eyes, in both tone and intensity. After years of observation and documentation, he emphatically states in his book, *The Elements of Colour*, that 'Every woman should know what colours are becoming to her; these will always be her subjective colours and their complements. . . .' So Itten concluded that our personal palette, the one to which we are drawn naturally, consists of the very colours that look best on us.

In adapting Itten's theory to fashion we have developed the four seasonal palettes as guides for clothing, makeup, and wardrobe planning. You don't have to be a brilliant colourist or fashion coordinator yourself, though you will look as if you are. Simply determine which

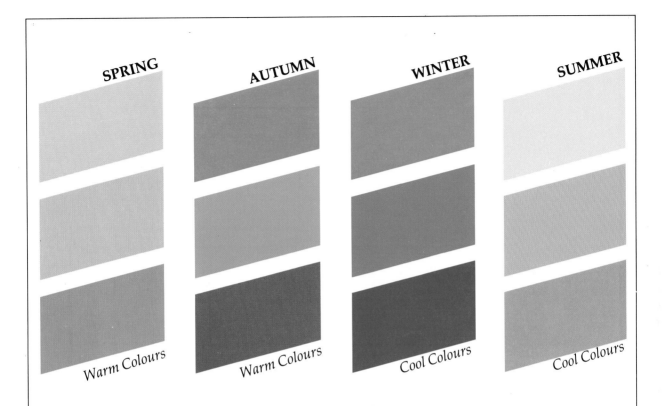

SPRING — *Warm Colours*

AUTUMN — *Warm Colours*

WINTER — *Cool Colours*

SUMMER — *Cool Colours*

You can wear almost any colour; it's the shade and intensity that count. Spring's colours are clear, delicate, or bright with yellow undertones. Autumn's colours are stronger with orange and gold undertones. Winter's colours are clear, vivid, or icy with blue undertones. And Summer's colours are cool and soft with blue undertones.

palette fits your colouring, wear those colours, and enjoy the compliments.

Perhaps the biggest joy in finding your personal colours is the freedom it brings. Using your colours, you will spend less time and energy shopping, yet you will have more confidence than ever that you look your best. Shopping will become quick and easy, because you will know what to look for and what to leave on the racks. You won't waste money or clutter up your wardrobe with mistakes. Your palette can be a tool that will simplify one aspect of your life, leaving you free to pursue other interests. It works for me. It works for others. It will work for you.

Betsy

Frances

WINTER

There are more Winters and they come in more varieties than any other seasonal type. Although their skin tones vary considerably, they all need the same cool, clear colours to look their best. Winters are the only ones who can wear black and pure white well. They come alive in true, vivid, and icy colours with a blue undertone.

Betsy has a pink skin tone, blue eyes with dark grey rims around the iris, and brown hair. Although her hair picks up some red highlights from the sun, its basic tone is ash brown. Compare these highlights with the true, metallic red tones in the hair of Autumn Laurie on page 48.

Frances's hair began to turn from black-brown to a silvery grey in her early twenties. Prematurely grey hair is most typical of Winters, and Winters tend to grey attractively, as you can see. Frances's skin tone is deep rose-beige and her eyes are a rosy brown.

Olive-skinned, dark-eyed and raven haired people are Winters. Although olive skin often appears golden, it actually has a blue undertone. Olive-skinned people and most blacks and Orientals look radiant in clear, vivid, cool colours, but sallow in warm colours. Most Winters have blue or brown eyes, but some have clear green, grey-green or hazel eyes with a grey tone. Young Winters often have light brown hair, though it usually darkens with age.

These colours are subject to the limitations of the printing process.

Pure White	Icy Green	Royal Blue	Shocking Pink
Light True Grey	Icy Yellow	Hot Turquoise	Deep Hot Pink
Medium True Grey	Icy Aqua	Chinese Blue	Magenta
Charcoal Grey	Icy Violet	Lemon Yellow	Fuchsia
Black	Icy Pink	Light True Green	Royal Purple
Grey-Beige (Taupe)	Icy Blue	True Green	Bright Burgundy
Navy Blue		Emerald Green	Blue-Red
True Blue	Silver-tone Accessories	Pine Green	True Red

Terry

SUMMER

Terry is a typical Summer with her rosy pink skin tone, blue eyes, and ash blonde hair. To keep the blonde look, Terry lightens her hair with an ash blonde rinse.

Katie's fair skin is almost translucent with a blue undertone. Her aqua-grey eyes change from blue to green, depending on what she is wearing.

Many Summers have freckles, eyes that are deep blue with white flecks, and hair that is medium brown. Summer is the only season who can successfully highlight her hair, because silver ash tones complement her blonde complexion.

Summer's eyes can also be green, hazel, or occasionally rosy brown. Most Summers have blonde, light brunette, or dark ash brown hair. The Summer is flattered by soft colours with a blue undertone. Note Katie's jacket is a soft white (not ivory), and Terry's blouse is a blue-pink rather than the coral pink worn by Susan, a Spring, on page 20.

Katie

These colours are subject to the limitations of the printing process.

Soft White

Powder Blue

Light Lemon Yellow

Lavender

Rose-Beige

Sky Blue

Powder Pink

Orchid

Cocoa

Medium Blue

Pastel Pink

Mauve

Rose-Brown

Periwinkle Blue

Rose Pink

Raspberry

Light Blue-Grey

Pastel Aqua

Deep Rose

Soft Fuchsia

Charcoal Blue-Grey

Pastel Blue-Green

Watermelon

Plum

Greyed Navy

Medium Blue-Green

Blue-Red

Silver-tone Accessories

Grey-Blue

Deep Blue-Green

Burgundy

AUTUMN

Colleen

Maura

Colleen has a true peach skin tone underneath those freckles. Her avocado green eyes and brown blonde hair make her an Autumn. Only an Autumn can look so lovely in pumpkin and olive green.

Maura's skin tone is ivory, and she is especially flattered by the muted Autumn tones, such as the bittersweet red turtleneck she is wearing under her oyster white jacket. Note the golden green colour of Maura's eyes and her golden brown hair, typical of the Autumn.

Most Autumns have brown, green or hazel eyes, but a few have bright turquoise eyes (usually the redheads). Autumn hair invariably has gold or red highlights, whether blonde, brunette, or vivid redhead. Carrot-coloured hair usually belongs to Autumns.

The Autumn is complemented by warm colours with golden undertones. Note that Laurie's lipstick (page 48) is brick red and her blouse is an orange-red rather than a blue-red.

These colours are subject to the limitations of the printing process.

Oyster White

Warm Beige

Coffee Brown

Dark Chocolate Brown

Mahogany

Camel

Gold

Medium Warm Bronze

Yellow-Gold

Mustard

Pumpkin

Terracotta

Rust

Deep Peach/Apricot

Salmon

Orange

Orange-Red

Bittersweet Red

Dark Tomato Red

Lime Green

Chartreuse

Bright Yellow-Green

Moss Green

Greyed Yellow-Green

Olive Green

Jade Green

Forest Green

Turquoise

Kingfisher Blue

Deep Periwinkle Blue

Gold-tone Accessories

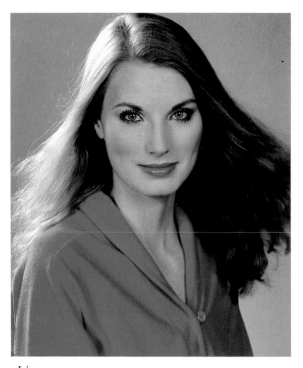

Lisa

SPRING

Lisa is a Spring with vivid red hair, and she looks especially good in her palette's brightest colours. Her fair ivory skin and pale blue eyes have a delicate quality, characteristic of many Springs.

Jennifer's ivory complexion looks like peaches and cream and is most flattered by Spring's softer colours, like the peach she is wearing. Her auburn blonde hair is characteristic of Spring, as are her deep blue eyes with their pale yellow flecks.

Holly (on page 48) is a typical Spring with her golden blonde hair, blue-green eyes, and peachy skin tone.

Though many Springs are blonde in childhood, their hair usually darkens with age, retaining its golden cast. Flaxen blondes, like Holly and Susan on pages 48 and 20, are the lucky ones who stay blonde naturally. Springs can have blue, green, hazel, or amber eyes, usually with golden tones. Notice that Spring Dorothy, on page 34, has blue eyes with a turquoise cast.

The Spring palette contains clear, warm colours, some delicate, some bright – all with yellow undertones. Note Holly's golden brown jacket on page 48. A darker brown is too harsh for her colouring.

Jennifer

These colours are subject to the limitations of the printing process.

Ivory

Light Clear Gold

Peach

Medium Violet

Buff

Bright Golden Yellow

Clear Salmon

Light Periwinkle Blue

Light Warm Beige

Pastel Yellow-Green

Bright Coral

Dark Periwinkle Blue

Camel

Medium Yellow-Green

Warm Pastel Pink

Light True Blue

Golden Tan (Honey)

Bright Yellow-Green

Coral Pink

Light Warm Aqua

Medium Golden Brown

Apricot

Clear Bright Warm Pink

Clear Bright Aqua

Light Warm Grey

Light Orange

Clear Bright Red

Medium Warm Turquoise

Light Clear Navy

Orange-Red

Gold-tone Accessories

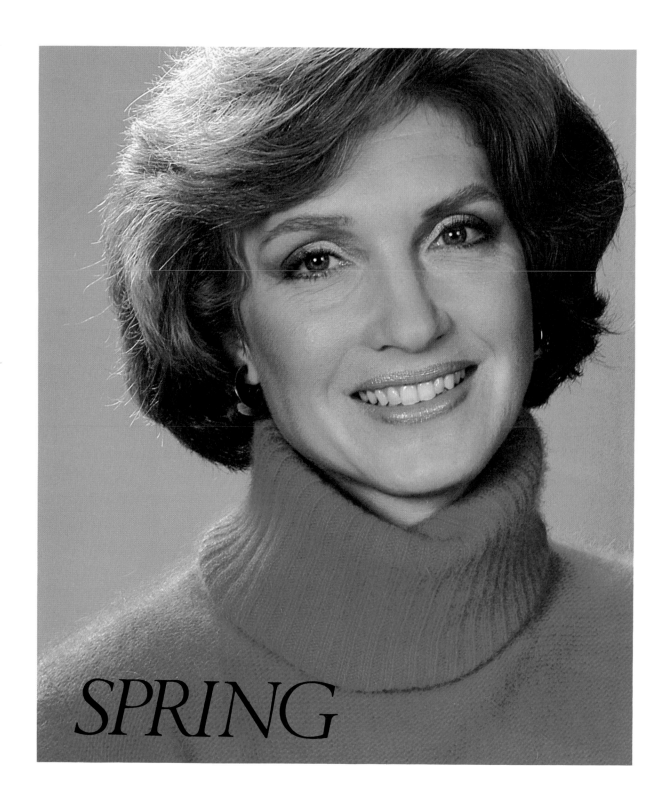

SPRING

CHAPTER FOUR

DETERMINING YOUR COLOURS:
The Colour Test

Now comes the fun – finding *your* colours! With these colours you can build a completely coordinated wardrobe, choose the right makeup, and create a new image that will truly reflect you.

The first step is to select key colours you have consistently worn with success throughout your lifetime. The second step is to evaluate your colouring – your skin, hair, and eyes. These two steps will tell you your season.

I am including a third optional step for those of you who would like to observe yourself in test colours, including makeup, the way we do in our classroom. This is best done in a group because it is difficult for people to see themselves objectively and other opinions are helpful. If you are already in a classroom situation, or perhaps a club, I strongly urge you to do Step 3 for the fun of it. It requires some effort to gather test colours, but the visual impact of seeing yourself and others in colours is most convincing!

STEP 1: YOUR COLOUR HISTORY

Select the group of colours below which you feel is most flattering to you, in general. As Johannes Itten proved with his art students, you will intuitively know whether you are better in cool or warm colours. The Summer and Winter palettes contain cool, blue-based colours; Autumn and Spring contain warm, yellow-based colours. Do not base your decision on the clothes currently hanging in your wardrobe. They may be right, but they may instead be the result of a current fad that is not necessarily for you! Pick the group containing the most colours that have brought you compliments all your life (even though you may be tired of wearing them). This test is based on comparison. Each column may have some colours that you have worn, but do they all look equally good on you? Ask yourself, 'Which group is *best*?'

Cool		Warm	
WINTER	*SUMMER*	*AUTUMN*	*SPRING*
Navy	Soft Blues	Dark Brown	Golden Brown
Black	Rose-Brown	Camel	Camel
White	Navy	Beige	Peachy Pink
Red	Rose Pink	Orange	Peach
Shocking Pink	Lavender	Gold	Soft Blues
Grey	Plum	Moss Green	Golden Yellow

Now look at the printed palette of your choice, as well as the charts on pages 58 to 61. Does the whole palette seem to suit you? If so, go on to Step 2. If not, make a second choice from the colour groups above, and then look at the palette for that season. If you are deciding between two seasons, ask yourself the following questions:

If you are deciding between

Winter and Autumn, ask: Am I better in navy, pure white, and clear colours (Winter) or brown, pumpkin, and muted gold (Autumn)? Be careful. Some brown-eyed Winters think they're Autumns. Brown is boring on a Winter, exciting on an Autumn. Ask your friends.

Winter and Summer, ask: Do I look good in pastels, like powder pink or blue (Summer), or do I need darker or brighter colours because pastels make me look washed out (Winter)?

Winter and Spring, ask: Am I really attractive in ivory, camel, and golden browns (Spring) or am I better in navy, pure white, and dark colours (Winter)?

Summer and Autumn, ask: Am I good in pastel blues and pinks but not in pumpkin or mustard colours (Summer) or is it the other way around (Autumn)?

Summer and Spring, ask:	Which do I wear better: buff, yellow-green, peachy pinks, golden browns (Spring) or blue-greens, blue-pinks, burgundy, or rose-tone browns (Summer)?
Spring and Autumn, ask:	Can I wear muted colours like mustard and moss green or very dark brown (Autumn) or am I better in clear colours like buff, light clear gold, peach, and lighter golden browns (Spring)? If neither seems quite right, try Summer. Many brown-eyed or green-eyed Summers mistakenly think they are warm seasons because they like camel, brown, and some greens. Summer has rose-brown, rose-beige, and many shades of blue-green.

Now pick your preferred season and move on to Step 2.

STEP 2: A LOOK AT YOUR COLOURING – THE SKIN TONE TEST

This step is to verify your selection in Step 1.

Take a long look at yourself in the mirror, near natural daylight if possible. Look at your skin, hair, and eyes, without makeup. If you colour your hair, try to remember its natural colour.

Your skin tone is the most important factor in determining the colours that look best on you. The tone of your skin comes from three pigments, melanin (brown), carotene (yellow), and hemoglobin (red). It is the particular combination of these three pigments that gives you your unique skin tone. Because your skin acts as a thin filter, it is the tone just under its surface that determines whether your colouring is cool or warm. Summers and Winters, the cool seasons, have blue undertones, while Autumns and Springs have golden undertones. Some people's skin tone is quite obvious, but for others the tone is subtle. In class, we compare wrists and palms. By comparison, you can often see whether you are more blue or golden than someone else. Take a piece of very white paper and hold it under your wrist and hand for comparison. Are you blue (or blue-pink) or are you golden (even orange)? If you have freckles, are they charcoal brown (cool) or golden brown (warm)?

Warning: Be careful not to confuse sallowness with a golden skin tone.

Anyone can have sallow skin, which appears yellow on the surface, regardless of its undertone. By the same token, any season can have a ruddy complexion, where the capillaries are close to the surface of the skin, giving an intense pinkness to the face. This should not necessarily be confused with a blue tone, as, ironically, ruddiness occurs most often in the warm seasons.

If you are uncertain of your skin tone, or if you are sallow or ruddy, look in the mirror at your entire body, nude, especially the untanned portions. Again, comparison is helpful. For example, my olive skin appears yellow at first glance, but in comparison to my daughter's ivory body, I look 'blue' and she looks 'golden.' She is an Autumn, I am a Winter.

Because your skin tone is not always obvious, here are more complete descriptions of the various types of colouring that typify each season, including hair and eyes. Read *only* the description of the season you selected in Step 1 and see if you find yourself. If you don't, then read the description of your second choice in Step 1. Combining your answers to Steps 1 and 2, pick whichever of these seasons you feel most suits you.

WINTER

Skin: First look for the blue or blue-pink undertone, but don't be discouraged if you can't readily see it. It's often subtle on a Winter. There are more Winters in the world than any other seasonal type. Winters may vary a great deal, yet they all need the same cool colours to look their best. The largest range of Winters are those with taupe-beige skin, ranging from light to dark, rosy or just plain beige. Most olive-skinned people, blacks, and Orientals are Winters, although a few are Autumns. Olive and Oriental skins can be confusing because they appear golden, as do the skins of some light blacks. But golden colours will make them appear sallow, while the cool Winter colours bring them to life. A Winter may also have milky white skin and dark hair (like Snow White). The white may have a visible pink tone or may appear pure white with a translucent quality. Winters do not usually have rosy cheeks, and their appearance improves dramatically with pink tone rouge or blusher.

Hair: Most Winters have dark hair, even though some were white-blonde in infancy. Brunette Winters have hair colour ranging from light brown to dark charcoal brown, sometimes with a touch of red highlights. Blue-black hair is typical of Winter, as is salt-and-pepper or silver grey. Of all the seasons, Winter is most likely to grey prematurely, and she often greys attractively. Rarely do we find a Winter who is naturally

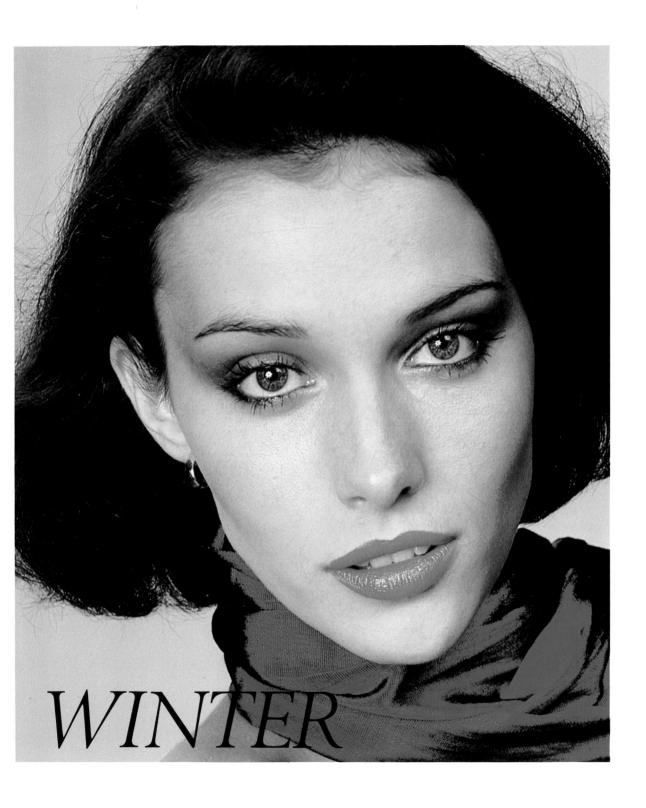

WINTER

blonde as an adult, but if she is, her hair is white-blonde, giving her a striking look.

Eyes: The Winter woman's eyes are most often a deep colour. They may be red-brown, black-brown, or hazel (a combination of grey-brown and blue or green); grey-blue, grey-green, or dark blue. The blue- or green-eyed Winter often has white flecks in the iris. Look closely at your eyes in a mirror and see, too, if they have a grey rim around the edge of the iris. Grey-rimmed eyes mean Winter or Summer, the cool seasons.

Well-known Winters: Elizabeth Taylor, Jacqueline Onassis, Audrey Hepburn, Cleo Laine, Shirley Bassey, Virginia Wade, Kiri te Kanawa.

Tick whichever characteristics describe you:

Skin: —Very white
—White with delicate pink tone
—Beige (no cheek colour, may be sallow)
—Rosy beige
—Olive
—Black (blue undertone)
—Charcoal-brown freckles

Hair: —Blue-black
—Medium brown (may have red highlights)
—Dark brown (taupe tone)
—Salt-and-pepper
—Silver-grey
—White blonde (rare)
—White

Eyes: —Dark red-brown
—Black-brown
—Hazel (grey-brown plus green or blue)
—Grey-blue
—Blue with white flecks in iris (may have grey rim)
—Dark blue
—Grey-green
—Green with white flecks in iris (may have grey rim)

SUMMER

Skin: Look for the blue undertone. Summers usually have visible pink in their skin. Some Summers are very fair and look pale without a little rouge. These fair Summers may have a translucent quality to the skin, and they are usually blonde, or were blonde in early childhood, and have light brown hair as they mature. Other Summers have very pink skin, with high colour, or rose-beige skin, ranging from fair to relatively deep rose-beige. A Summer may be sallow, especially on her arms, but there is usually visible pink in her cheeks.

Hair: As a child, Summer is most often blonde, ranging from a towhead to ash blonde to dark ash. As she matures, her hair tends to darken to a 'mousy' colour, so named because of its greyish cast. Brunette Summers also have hair colour ranging from light to dark brown, again with ash overtones. Occasionally a Summer has auburn highlights in her hair, especially if she gets lots of sun. The Summer woman greys gracefully to a blue-grey or pearly white tone. Summers, of all the seasons, most often feel the need to 'brighten' themselves with hair colour or highlighting. A Summer woman truly benefits from wearing her colours, as her colours alone bring 'life' to her face.

Eyes: Summer eyes are most often blue, green, aqua, or soft hazel (predominantly blue or green with greyed brown surrounding the pupil). The Summer eye often has a cloudy look inside the iris, rather than a clear, transparent colour. Many Summers have soft grey eyes or eyes with a grey rim around the iris, and white flecks in an irregular pattern inside the iris. And intensely blue eyes are characteristic of some lucky Summers. A few Summers have soft brown eyes.

Well-known Summers: Queen Elizabeth II, the Princess of Wales, Susannah York, Penelope Keith, Julie Christie, the late Princess Grace of Monaco.

Tick whichever characteristics describe you:

Skin: —Pale beige with delicate pink cheeks
     —Pale beige with no cheek colour (even sallow)
     —Very pink
     —Rosy or charcoal brown freckles

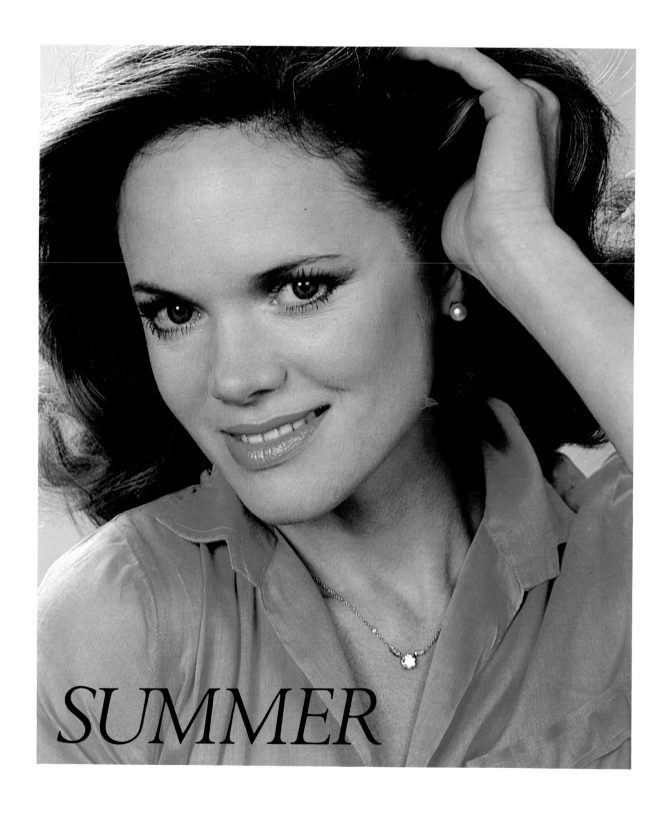

SUMMER

Hair: —Platinum blonde
　　　—Ash blonde (often towhead as a child)
　　　—'Mouse' blonde
　　　—'Mouse' brown
　　　—Dark brown (taupe tone)
　　　—Brown with auburn cast
　　　—Blue-grey

Eyes: —Blue (with brown around pupil and 'cloudy' iris, grey rim)
　　　—Grey-blue
　　　—Grey-green
　　　—Pale grey
　　　—Blue with white flecks (may have grey rim)
　　　—Green with white flecks (may have grey rim)
　　　—Hazel (blue and brown or green and brown)
　　　—Bright, clear blue
　　　—Clear, pale aqua (eyes change from blue to green, depending on clothes)
　　　—Soft brown

AUTUMN

Skin: Look for the golden undertone. Even a ruddy Autumn is more 'orange' than 'blue'. The Autumn comes in three varieties: the fair person with ivory or creamy peach skin; the true redhead, fair to dark, often with freckles; and the golden-beige brunette, whose skin ranges from medium to deep copper, the latter having charcoal black hair. Many Autumns are pale or sallow and especially need an orange-tone rouge to 'come alive'. An Autumn and a Spring may have similar colouring, but the Autumn will usually have colourless cheeks, while Spring's cheeks will be rosy. A few Orientals and blacks are Autumns, if they have a truly golden undertone, but most are Winters.

Hair: Autumn can be golden blonde as a child, usually darkening as she matures. Redheads, ranging from carrot to those with auburn or red-brown hair, are usually Autumns. (A few redheads are Springs, having colouring too delicate to handle the stronger Autumn palette.) Many Autumns are brunette, their hair usually having a gold or metallic red cast. Occasionally, an Autumn has charcoal black hair. An Autumn should cover grey, as it tends to come in yellow-grey, and the two-tone look is drab on her, especially if she's a redhead. However, once her hair is completely grey, it can be most attractive.

Eyes: Most Autumns have brown or green eyes. Their brown eyes are dark to topaz, and their green eyes often sport gold or brown flecks in the iris. Isolated flecks, either gold, brown, or black, are often present in the Autumn eye. Some Autumns have clear green eyes, like glass, or deep olive green 'cat' eyes. An Autumn's hazel eye contains golden brown, green, and gold. A few Autumns have vivid turquoise or aqua eyes, but not a true blue or grey-blue eye colour.

Well-known Autumns: Vanessa Redgrave, Carol Burnett, Shirley MacLaine, Katharine Hepburn, Lucille Ball, Maggie Smith, Glenda Jackson.

Tick whichever characteristics describe you:

Skin: —Ivory
  —Ivory with freckles (usually redhead)
  —Peach
  —Peach with freckles (usually golden blonde, brown)
  —Golden beige (no cheek colour, needs rouge)
  —Dark beige (coppery)
  —Golden black

Hair: —Red
  —Coppery red-brown
  —Chestnut brown
  —Golden brown
  —Golden blonde
  —Charcoal black
  —Golden grey

Eyes: —Dark brown
  —Golden brown
  —Amber
  —Hazel (golden brown, green gold)
  —Green (with brown or gold flecks)
  —Pale, clear green
  —Blue with a distinct aqua or turquoise tone

SPRING

Skin: Look for the golden undertone. Springs have the most delicate quality of all the seasonal types. Spring's skin is either creamy ivory, peachy pink, or peach-beige. Freckles come naturally to her, though some Springs have skin clear as glass, often called 'peaches and cream'. The ivory Spring appears to have golden flecks or highlights to her skin, while the peachy Spring is likely to have peachy pink cheeks. Of all the seasons, Springs are the most likely to have rosy cheeks and to flush easily. Their skin is usually finely textured, and colour seems to rush to the surface. Some Springs are very ruddy and can be confused with Summers because of this apparent pinkness. Look at the parts of your body that don't blush to see whether you are peach or truly pink. Springs have an aliveness and brightness to their skin tone, even if they are extremely fair.

Hair: Spring's hair is golden blonde, strawberry, bright red, or golden brown. Ash-tone hair is not Spring. In childhood many Springs are blonde, ranging from flaxen to honey to strawberry, but their hair often darkens with age. Some have very dark brown hair. A few Springs have vivid carrot-red hair, missing being Autumns by their need for clear colours. Grey does not arrive gracefully on Spring, so she is wise to keep her hair dyed its youthful colour.

Eyes: Spring's eyes are most often blue, green, or aqua. Some have eyes as clear as glass. Others have a golden cluster surrounding the pupil. Many Springs have blue eyes that appear to be a solid steel grey from a distance, but up close, they are really blue and have a sunburst of white 'rays' coming from the pupil. There are some brown-eyed Springs, but they are always golden brown or topaz. A Spring's hazel eye contains golden brown, green, and gold.

Well-known Springs: Zsa Zsa and Eva Gabor, Debbie Reynolds, Julie Andrews, Marilyn Monroe, Margaret Thatcher, Nancy Reagan.

Tick whichever characteristics describe you:

Skin: —Ivory
      —Ivory with pale golden freckles
      —Peach
      —Golden beige
      —Rosy cheeks

Hair: —Flaxen blonde
      —Golden blonde
      —Strawberry blonde (usually with freckles)
      —Strawberry redhead (usually with freckles)
      —Auburn
      —Golden brown
      —Red-black (rare)
      —Golden grey

Eyes: —Blue with white 'rays' (appear steel grey from distance)
      —Clear blue (may have brown flecks)
      —Clear green (may have golden flecks)
      —Aqua
      —Bright blue with turquoise tone
      —Light golden brown

By now you should know your season. If you want to verify your choice, or if you are still deciding between two seasons, take Step 3 and see yourself in colours. Otherwise, move on and begin putting your colours to use.

The only trick now is emotionally accepting your whole palette – both the colours that are new for you and the missing colours that you have previously worn. The missing colours are gone for two reasons – they upset your wardrobe plan, including your makeup and accessories, and they don't look as good on you as the colours in your palette. Once your eye is adjusted to you in your palette, you will be the first to see that the 'old' colour doesn't look that good after all. Be open-minded, too, about the new colours in your palette. In class, both the students and I are a support system to convince a hesitant Summer that she really does look great in her fuchsia, or a red-headed Autumn that she can wear red, now that it's the right red.

Now have fun learning more about your colour personality. But don't go on a major shopping spree until you've read the rest of the book. You want to be a totally harmonious woman, with your wardrobe, accessories, hair, and makeup just right, before you go out and set the world on fire!

STEP 3: (OPTIONAL): SEEING YOURSELF IN TEST COLOURS

First you will try yourself in makeup colours and then you'll drape your neck and shoulders in fabric colours to see which colours bring out the best in you.

MAKEUP TEST

Trying on lipstick and rouge colours from opposite seasons is the quickest way to reveal whether your skin tone is warm or cool. You may use lip gloss and any type of blusher on your cheeks. Even if you prefer not to wear makeup, this test is invaluable in helping you accurately determine your season. Because *many* of the women who come to my classes are wearing the wrong colour lipstick, and because your eye is accustomed to seeing whatever makeup you have been wearing to date, you may want to ask a friend or a salesperson to help.

When you try on these colours, wear an off-white shirt or something in a pale neutral so your eye will not judge the colour in relation to your clothing. Do not wear any foundation on your face, as you want your skin to show its natural tone.

Now try on the lip and cheek colours that apply to the seasons in question for you. Most department stores or chemists' shops have plenty of testers available, or perhaps you have some of these colours floating around your household. Use the following chart as a guide:

		Lipstick	*Rouge*
For the Cool Seasons	WINTER	Medium to Dark Pink/Plum or True Red (no orange tones)	Burgundy or Plum
	SUMMER	Light to Medium Pink	Plum or Pink
For the Warm Seasons	AUTUMN	Orange or Mocha	Dark Peach or Russet
	SPRING	Light Peach, Coral, or Coral-Pink	Peach

WINTER

Trena

SUMMER

Barbara

SPRING

Holly

AUTUMN

Laurie

When you study what each lipstick/rouge combination does to your skin, always *compare*. One colour may look good, but its opposite may look *better*.

The Winter usually needs colour and will look decidedly better in pink or plum than in orange tones. Olive-skinned Winters may be accustomed to wearing peach, but try a deep pink and see the difference! Autumn is the only one who will look good in orange. Summer will usually find the Winter tester too strong, though not always. But she will definitely look better in either of the pink testers than in the orange. She will not look terrible in Spring's peach, but she will look better in pink. Spring wears a peach or coral best of all. Autumn's orange will be too harsh and muted for Spring, even though it is a warm colour.

FABRIC TEST

Now it's time to see yourself draped in colours. A solid colour scarf, blouse, sheet, towel, or even paper will do. Avoid prints. Use the colours of the printed palettes as guides.

This test is based on comparison. You should compare one colour against another, perhaps several times, to see which is better. You may need to compare several sets of colours until you get a clear feeling for the season that is most in harmony with you.

First, there are a few rules you should follow to make the test accurate.

1. Find a place with plenty of natural daylight. You can't see the subtleties of colour in dim lighting or under fluorescent light. (I am often asked by well-meaning people to analyse their season at a party over candlelight. Alas, only a magician can do this trick!)

2. Cover your clothes with a large white shirt or sheet. It is extremely distracting for the untrained eye to judge one colour while another colour is competing for attention.

3. If you dye or colour your hair in any way, cover it with an off-white scarf. The eye will look at colour plus hair, rather than colour plus skin. You want to see what the test colours do to your skin only. Most people who have trouble determining a season are those whose hair is coloured or highlighted. (There's no harm in trying on wigs, if you can find any. I keep four on hand in many classroom: neutral brown for Winters and brunette Summers, auburn for Autumns and Springs, ash blonde for blonde Summers, and golden blonde for Springs.)

4. Ask at least two other people (preferably three or four) to do this test with you. One person is not enough because her (or his) opinion may be influenced by personal colour preferences rather than by how the colour looks on you. Undoubtedly you have colleagues, neighbours, friends, or family who can spare a few minutes to share opinions. (If you must do this test by yourself in front of a mirror, then switch the colours back and forth, allowing each to settle for a minute until you have a clear feeling which group is best.)

5. Gather whichever colours you need to make your comparisons. Use the printed colours on pages 27 to 33 as guidelines.

6. Try to divorce yourselves from your personal favourite and least favourite colours while observing each other. You are not judging the colour, but rather its effectiveness in revealing skin tone. When holding the test colours under your face, you must remember one all-important rule: *LOOK AT THE FACE, NOT AT THE COLOUR.*

Remember, this is a test based on comparison. One colour may look good, but its opposite may look better. Always ask, 'Which is better?'

Here's what you look for as you hold a colour to your face:

The Right Colour:	The Wrong Colour:
Smoothes and clarifies your complexion; minimises lines, shadows, and circles; brings a healthy colour to your face. Your face will pop out, pushing the colour into the background.	May make your complexion look pale, sallow, or 'muddy'; will accentuate lines or shadows around the mouth and nose, dark circles under the eyes; will accentuate blotches, if any; may age your face; will look too strong or too weak. The colour tends to pop out, pushing your face into the background.

Now compare the colours of the two seasons you have picked from Steps 1 and 2. If you are deciding between a warm and a cool season you must do the test without lipstick or your eye will be influenced by the colour on your lips.

AUTUMN or WINTER
Orange-Red or Blue-Red
Warm Beige or Pure White
Dark Brown or Navy Blue
Orange or Magenta

AUTUMN or SPRING
Mustard or Light Clear Gold
Dark Brown or Golden Brown
Bright Orange or Light Peach
Moss Green or Pastel
Yellow-Green

AUTUMN or SUMMER
Orange-Red or Blue-Red
Camel or Rose-Brown
Orange or Powder Pink
Moss Green or Blue-Green

SUMMER or SPRING
Blue-Red or Orange-Red
Rose-Brown or Golden Brown
Blue-Green or Yellow-Green
Rose-Pink (Blue) or Peach

SUMMER or WINTER
Rose-Brown or Black (with
    makeup)
Soft White or Pure White
Powder Pink or Magenta
Soft Blue or Royal Blue

WINTER or SPRING
Blue-Red or Orange-Red
Pure White or Ivory
Black or Camel
Magenta or Peach

Now, try out your season by wearing something you already own in one of your season's colours, being careful to use the appropriate make-up shades. Go out somewhere so that your friends and acquaintances can see you. Their compliments will confirm your choice!

CHAPTER FIVE

YOUR COLOUR PERSONALITY
Understanding Your Palette

I once met a delicate Spring, of grandmotherly age yet retaining a youthful quality as Springs often do. She appeared at her first session of my class in powder blue, looking soft, feminine, and dainty, entirely in tune with her personality even though powder blue was not her perfect colour. After receiving her spring colours, she returned to class the following week in a wild Indian print dress sporting every bright colour in the spring palette! She had clearly misinterpreted her colours.

Your colours work best when you use them to harmonise with your colouring, your body type, and your personality. Our Spring, for example, with her flaxen hair, pale blue eyes, and ivory complexion, had a soft appearance. To achieve her best look, she needed to build her wardrobe around her delicate to medium colours, using only the merest touches of bright as accents. The geometric Indian print was out of character for her.

Within your palette you must choose the colours and combinations that suit you as an individual. Each of the palettes contains both soft and vivid colours, all of which are valuable to you in planning your wardrobe. But some of you may feel most comfortable with a soft image; others may love their bright colours best; and still others prefer to dress in neutrals. Further, your moods may change from year to year. So use your palette to reflect your own personality, knowing that all your colours are flattering.

Bear in mind, too, that the colouring of people within each season varies in intensity. Most people wear all their colours well, but some, depending on their hair colour or the depth of their skin tone, wear some colours best near the face, saving others for accessories or clothing further from the face. If you are quite fair, for example, you may find that a few of the brightest or darkest colours in your palette are too strong to wear in a large splash near your face. You can still wear these colours, but you should use them in prints, accents, skirts, trousers, or accessories. A jacket in one of your dark or bright colours would look best if softened by a blouse in a lighter shade. In contrast, the woman with stronger colouring may find her palest colours or neutrals a little weak, and she should keep her brightest shades near her face and the softer ones in the jacket, skirt, or accessories. With a suntan, a fair person can usually wear her vivid colours.

TRYING YOUR COLOURS

Now it's time to try on your colours and decide how to use them to your best advantage. Begin by cutting out the printed swatches for your season and placing them in a plastic wallet to keep safely tucked in your handbag. The neutrals are arranged together, and the colour families are together. Now go on a looking spree, not to buy, but to hold up colours to yourself. Start with your own wardrobe, your family's clothes, and then the shops. Remember, at this point you are just looking in order to understand your colour 'personality'.

Pay special attention to your neutral and basic colours. These will become the backbone of your wardrobe, as they are the ones you will use for a basic coat, suit, and dress. You will usually find some of your neutrals more exciting than others, depending on your hair and eye colour. A grey-haired Winter, for example, is especially attractive in a grey coat, while a brunette may be better in navy, using her grey for trousers and skirts. When her hair turns grey, she can switch.

You will not find all your colours at once. The fashion industry promotes some colours every year, but most come in cycles. Also, your season's colours are usually easiest to find during 'your' season, as this is when these colours fill the shops. But your colours last a lifetime, so eventually you'll have an opportunity to try them all. As I mentioned earlier, your skin tone doesn't change, but it does fade with age. You will not change your palette, but you will draw from your own softer colours once you've become a great-grandmother. By the same token, if you are sixteen, you may want to save your sophisticated shades for later. You are lucky to find your colours so young!

The colours you are trying on will always look best when you are wearing the correct makeup. Even if you dislike makeup, I strongly suggest that you wear blusher. It can be applied to look natural, and you will look healthier and prettier with a little colour on your cheeks.

As you 'colour shop', try to develop an impression of your colour self in your mind. Familiarise yourself thoroughly with your colours so that when you shop later for clothes, you will understand your palette. In the future, a 'new' colour may appear on the fashion scene, one that is not printed in your palette. When you've lived in your palette a while, you will know when a new fashion colour is for you.

The charts on pages 58 to 61 and the descriptions that follow are to be used along with your printed swatches to help you to conceptualise your season. These are your guidelines when you shop 'for real' later.

The swatches themselves are to be used as a guide, not as an absolute. Colour printed on paper is less true than colour in fabric. You do not have to match the swatches exactly, except where specifically mentioned in the following descriptions. For most colours, you may use your range of, say, greens, held against the garment in question to see if it blends. If it doesn't, it's not for you.

WINTER

You are best in clear colours and sharp contrasts. A Winter strives to stay snappy and should *never* wear muted, powdered tones. When shopping, think *true, blue* and *vivid; sharp, clear,* and *icy.*

Winter is the only season who successfully wears pure white or black. Don't be afraid of a white blouse; white is exciting on you. Winter's greys range from icy to charcoal; and true grey is yours, but not blue-grey or yellow-grey. Your beige *must* be taupe (grey-beige), always light and clear. You are not a beige person in general and should avoid all rose-beiges and yellow-beiges. Darker taupe may be used for accessories such as shoes and bags. Navy blue is excellent on you, as is burgundy. You may wear any shade of navy, but keep your burgundy bright. You will not look your best in muted maroon tones.

Winter excels in true and primary colours, as well as their bluer and darker counterparts. You wear true red and any blue-red, but not orange-red. Your greens range from true green to emerald to pine, which has a blue cast rather than the yellow cast of Autumn's forest green. True blue, royal blue, hot turquoise, and Chinese blue as well as navy make up your blue family. Royal purple is great, as are hot pinks, from shocking pink to magenta to fuchsia. You have only one shade of yellow: clear, bright lemon. Avoid golden yellow.

Icy tones make the Winter woman sparkle. These are your version of pastels, almost white with a drop of colour. You wear icy blue, icy aqua, icy pink, icy violet, icy green, and icy yellow as well as icy versions of your other colours, such as grey and taupe. Avoid all powdered pastels, as they will dull you.

The very fair-skinned Winter is best in the icy and deep colours. The shocking colours are too vivid in large amounts, and she should wear them as accents or away from the face. Deep hot pink, for example, will be better on her than shocking pink. True emerald, or pine green is better than light true green; blue-red and burgundy are better than true red, and so forth. Fair Winters may also find soft white better than pure white and should soften black near the face. They should mix black with other colours, or wear a scoop neck, letting their skin do the softening. By contrast, some Winters are especially good in the true, bright colours and weak in the palest neutrals, such as grey and beige. Such Winters should use these neutrals in prints or mix them with a brighter colour near the face.

If you are a Winter you should never wear orange, gold, rust, peach, orange-reds, yellow-greens, or most beiges and browns. You may wear brown if it is so dark that it can be worn with black accessories. Avoid all muted, dull tones. Stick closely to your colour swatches when shopping for your yellow and your taupe. You may deviate from the other swatches up or down a shade.

SUMMER

Summer is the pastel woman and the woman who wears soft neutrals especially well. You should think *blue, rose,* and *soft.* Even though you may be a Summer who favours her bright colours, you should think of yourself as feminine, looking more for softness than for sharp contrast. On you the pastels look strong and vibrant enough.

Soft white (with no yellow) is Summer's best white. Ironically, this is the shade called 'winter white' in the shops. Your beige and brown always have a rose tone. Wear any shade between your rose-beige and rose-brown swatches, including cocoa, but avoid yellow-beiges, grey-beiges, and dark browns. You can wear greys from very light blue-grey to any soft charcoal blue-grey.

You are in your territory in most blues, eliminating only the royal or Chinese shades of Winter. Your swatches for blues are simply guides. Keep your aqua light to medium, and your navy greyer and softer than the strong navy of Winter. Greyed navy brings out the beauty of your softer complexion. Blue-greens, ranging from pastel to deep, also belong to Summer, as do all pastel pinks with a blue undertone. You may carry your pinks into deep rose tones, including fuchsia, but often they are best when powdered or muted. Your reds, like your greys and greens, have blue tones. Your watermelon leans a bit toward coral, but you should avoid orange or orange-reds.

The whole family of lavender, orchid, and mauve pastels belongs to Summer. All of them are for you. In addition, you have the darker tones of plum, burgundy, and raspberry, though fair Summers may need to keep a softer shade near the face.

Summer has only one flattering shade of yellow: light lemon. You should stick closely to your yellow swatch and avoid gold tones.

The very fair blonde Summer should soften her darkest colours, such as plum, dark burgundy, and maroon with a lighter colour close to her face. The dark brunette Summer is especially good in the vivid colours of her palette and may find that the palest pastels are best mixed with brighter colours. She is the woman who just missed being a Winter.

All Summers should avoid black, pure white, yellow-beige, gold, orange, yellow-greens, and all yellow undertones. Black may be used as an accessory in shoes and bags. With a tan, a Summer woman may get away with pure white, but it is still too strong a look for your overal soft image. You do not want to look sharp around the edges.

AUTUMN

You Autumns have the easiest shopping! Your colours are readily available. And because you can wear either muted or clear tones, you needn't be too careful in matching your swatches. You may use your swatches as a general guide, except for your blues, where you should stick to your printed samples. Always think of golden undertones when you shop.

Your best white is oyster, a beige-tone white. You wear all warm beiges, from light to dark, except taupe (grey-beige) and rose-beige. Dark chocolate brown is especially exciting on you, though you wear all browns well – mahogany, camel, tan, and bronze tones. Any gold, yellow-gold, pumpkin, mustard, or terracotta is good. Your oranges range from medium peach and muted salmon to bright orange and rust. Orange-reds and bittersweet reds are your best. Yellow-greens, from greyed to bright, and earth greens, from jade to moss, are for you. Forest green is especially becoming. Be careful with your blues. Your turquoise and kingfisher blue are strong and muted, and your periwinkle is deep.

The very fair Autumn may be overwhelmed by the strength of the brightest colours, such as orange, chartreuse, bright yellow-green, and turquoise. She is best in the soft or muted colours, the neutrals, peach, periwinkle, and jade. By contrast, a dark-skinned Autumn may look a little drab in the muted earth colours of this palette. She needs to wear her bright colours closest to her face, saving the muted ones for skirts and shoes, or to mix in prints. She needs makeup to look her best in beige and softer colours.

All Autumns should avoid black, pink, navy, grey, blue-reds, and all colours with blue undertones. Be careful that your peach, periwinkle, and lime green are not too pale.

SPRING

Springs are the most delicate of all the seasons, yet they need colours that are alive. When you shop, think *clear, warm* (yellow), and *crisp.* Your colours are the hardest to find, because they must be clear, never muted, and not too dark. Because of your delicate beauty, you remain ageless – a compensation for having to search a little harder for your colours.

Spring's best white is ivory, a creamy tone, though you may also wear off-white. Your beiges are all clear and warm – from light beige to camel. Your browns begin with golden tan and go as dark as milk chocolate; any golden brown is good as long as it is not too dark. Spring has clear golds, from buff to golden yellow, bright but not harsh.

Only one shade of grey is flattering to Spring: warm (yellow) grey, in a light shade if near the face. Spring's navy blue is light navy, clear and bright. Dark navy is harsh and ageing. Stick closely to your swatches.

Spring has many shades of aqua and clear turquoise, and these are especially good on you. You are also vibrant in light true blue, periwinkle blue, from light to dark, and medium violet. Although Spring is often accustomed to wearing powder blue, you are not as exciting in it as you are in your periwinkle shades.

Peach, apricot, salmon, and coral, as well as all peachy pinks, are for Spring. You may wear any light orange, bright coral, and orange-red. You are good in clear red, but must avoid blue-reds. Yellow-greens are for you as long as they are clear. Your greens range from pastel to bright.

The very fair, delicate Spring is overpowered by too much of her brightest colours, such as bright golden yellow, bright yellow-green, and sometimes clear red and violet. For her, these are accent colours, good as a sash around a sun hat or in beach clothes or funwear. By contrast, the Spring with stronger colouring looks great in a whole dress of bright yellow-green or golden yellow, but she looks pale in her lightest colours and sometimes in camel. These are best when mixed or used as accessories. This Spring may also add a clear, light rust, and a bright, clear kingfisher or peacock blue to her palette.

Avoid black, pure white, colours with blue undertones, dark and muted colours, but you may wear black in prints, unless you are very fair.

COMPARISON OF THE COLOURS OF THE FOUR SEASONAL PALETTES

	WINTER	SUMMER
White	Pure White	Soft White
Beige	Grey-Beige (Taupe) Icy Taupe	Rose-Beiges

Grey	True Greys, from Icy
	    to Charcoal
		Blue-Greys,
		    Light to Medium

Brown	No Brown No Tan	Rose-Browns Cocoa
Black	Black	No Black
Navy	Any Navy	Greyed Navy
Blue	True Blue Royal Blue Icy Blue	Grey-Blue (including Denim) Sky Blue Periwinkle Blue Powder to Medium Blue
Turquoise	Hot Turquoise Chinese Blue Icy Aqua	Pastel Aqua
Green	Light True Green True Green Emerald Green Icy Green	Blue-Greens, Pastel to Deep

	AUTUMN	SPRING
White	Oyster White	Ivory

Beige	Earth Beiges
	Gold-tone Beiges,
	   including Camel
		Clear Beiges
		Creamy Beiges, including
		   Camel

Grey	No Grey	Warm (Yellow) Greys, Light to Medium

Brown	Dark Brown,
	   Most Browns, Tans
	   Coffee, Mahogany,
	   Bronze
		Golden Browns,
		   Clear Tans

Black	No Black	No Black
Navy	No Navy	Light Clear Navy
Blue	Kingfisher Blue Deep Periwinkle	Light Royal Blue Periwinkle Blues, Light to Dark
Turquoise	Turquoise	Medium Warm Turquoise Clear Aquas

Green	Grey Yellow-Greens
	Yellow-Greens,
	   Lime to Bright
	Earth Greens,
	   Olive, Moss, Jade,
	Forest
		Clear Yellow-Greens,
		   Pastel to Bright

COMPARISON OF THE COLOURS OF THE FOUR SEASONAL PALETTES

	WINTER	SUMMER
Orange	No Orange	No Orange
Pink	Shocking Pink Deep Hot Pink (Blue) Magenta, Fuchsia Icy Pink	All Pastel Pinks (Blue) Deep Rose Blue-Pinks
Red	True Red Blue-Reds	Watermelon Blue-Reds Raspberry

Burgundy	Bright Burgundy	Burgundy,
		  including Maroons
		  and Red Browns

Gold	No Gold	No Gold
Yellow	Clear Lemon Yellow Icy Yellow	Light Lemon Yellow
Purple	Royal Purple Icy Violet	Plum Soft Fuchsia Mauve, Orchid, Lavender

	AUTUMN	**SPRING**
Orange	All Oranges Deep Peach, Salmon Rust, Terracotta	Light Oranges Apricot, Peach, Salmon All Corals, Light Rust
Pink	No Pink	All Peachy (Yellow) Pinks
Red	Orange-Reds Bittersweet Dark Tomato	Clear Red Orange-Reds
Burgundy	No Burgundy	No Burgundy
Gold	All Golds	Clear Gold
Yellow	Yellow-Gold	Bright Golden Yellow
Purple	No Purple	Medium Violet Blue-Violet

COMMONLY ASKED QUESTIONS

There are three questions I am inevitably asked in my classes:

1. *Could I be more than one season?*

The answer is no. You will look *best* in one palette; your wardrobe coordinates in one palette; and your makeup goes with one palette. Further, each palette has its own personality. As you grow into your season you develop a special image. You will defeat the purpose of your colours if you adopt two seasons.

Occasionally a woman of redheaded complexion can combine the Autumn and Spring colours, removing colours that are too strong or those that clash with her hair. Her makeup and accessories will blend because the seasons are both warm. She should call herself an Autumn, even though she will be wearing some Spring colours.

2. *Why can't I wear black if I'm not a Winter?*

Black is too strong for all but a Winter. Blonde hair will look blonder, but your face will be overpowered and less beautiful in black. People will see your blonde hair and black dress before they notice *you*. If black turns you on, why not wear it in the bedroom? It's a wonderfully sexy colour.

3. *What if I'm in the wrong season?*

You'll know very quickly. Mistakes usually occur only on the person who colours or highlights her hair.

Wear the colours of the season you think you are for one week, drawing from clothes you already own and using the appropriate makeup. Listen for compliments and ask your friends. If it isn't working, do the same with your second season. If you colour your hair, go to a wig department, and try on different hair colours.

Repeat the original test if necessary, including Step 3.

Now that you know your colour personality and understand your palette, let's move on to your clothing personality. Your colours and your type are the most important aspects of selecting clothing to express and complement the real you.

CHAPTER SIX

YOUR CLOTHING PERSONALITY
What Type Are You?

What word comes to mind when you think of the following movie and stage personalities? Shirley Bassey, Carol Burnett, Sandy Duncan, Liz Taylor? For me, Shirley Bassey is dramatic; Carol Burnett, funny and down-to-earth; Sandy Duncan, a pixie; Liz Taylor, sexy. Perhaps you have different reactions, but you will probably agree that each of these women has a type. Picture Shirley Bassey in a dramatic halter-top gown with a diamond-shaped cutout exposing her navel. Looks terrific – on her. Now imagine Carol Burnett appearing in the same gown. Ridiculous? Of course. And wouldn't Sandy Duncan look out of character in Elizabeth Taylor's low-cut satin?

Your clothing personality – the type or 'flavour' in clothing that is best for you – is partially determined by your season because your palette has a certain personality of its own.

A Winter, with her dark (or white) hair and deep eyes, tends towards the dramatic. Looking at the Winter palette, you can see that these colours have a dramatic, sophisticated, perhaps formal, quality, calling for clothes with sleek, clean lines. Her prints must have value contrast and are best worn away from the face, with the exception of small scarves. The Winter is usually best in solids, for her palette's striking colours speak for themselves.

The Summer palette has classic colours, reflecting calmness and conservatism, and the Summer woman is most often a poised, gracious, even-tempered person, ideal in classic clothes and soft prints. She's the elegant, but feminine type.

Autumn's palette speaks of warmth and friendliness. The Autumn woman is probably the natural, informal person, best in casual, sporty clothes. She's good in paisleys, tweeds, and casual, colourful prints.

The colours in Spring's palette are lively, bright, and youthful. Spring herself is often a friendly, informal, bubbly person who never seems to age and has a girlish, feminine quality even in her clothes. Her prints are crisp and colourful, but delicate in feeling.

But what if you are a Winter who is tiny, with rounded features and an innocent, youthful quality – not dramatic at all? Or perhaps you're a Spring who is five feet nine inches tall, with an athletic build, captain of the local hockey team. You may have the delicate, youthful colouring of a Spring, but you certainly would not look your best dressed in girlish ruffles.

Determining the personality in clothing that best suits you depends on more than your season. Your type derives, in addition, from your facial features, height, and bone structure.

It's time to study yourself in the mirror again, this time in a full-length mirror. If you don't have one, put it on your priority list. A full-length mirror is your most honest friend and the only way to get a realistic view of yourself.

Stand in front of the mirror and look first at your face. Do you have even, regular features or a prominent nose or chin or perhaps high cheekbones? Do you have a square jaw? Big eyes? A turned-up nose?

Now check out your body. Is your neck long, short, or average? Are your shoulders square, sloped, or average? Are they broad or narrow? Are you buxom or flat or somewhere in the middle? Is your waist anything special in either direction? How about your hips? Round? Flat? Are your legs long, short, average?

Let's see how your body and features help you arrive at the best look for you. The sooner you understand and accept your body type, the happier you will be. Trying to wear high-style, boy-cut clothes when your figure is shaped like an hourglass only results in disappointment. You will look your best when you dress to enhance what you are instead of trying to be what you are not. Make the most of your uniqueness!

FASHION TYPES

To illustrate the differences among types, we'll identify dramatic, sporty/natural, romantic, ingenue, and classic. In addition, we'll take a look at business wear for all types. These images are not absolutes and they may overlap, but you will see how each type influences the selection of clothes, makeup, hair style, and accessories.

DRAMATIC

The woman who wears the dramatic look well is usually tall and thin, with dark or striking colouring and angular features. Any sharp or prominent facial feature is great on a dramatic. So are broad, even bony, shoulders. (See how you can turn your least favourite qualities into assets?) If you aren't tall, but have dramatic features, you may dress dramatically in touches, but not all over. Full-fledged dramatics are skinny and exotic-looking and have flat hips and long legs.

The dramatic type wears extremes in fashion – either straight lines and hard-finish fabrics or ultra billowy clothes. If you are dramatic, you may wear severely plain or lavishly ornate fabrics and styles. Wear the most exotic colours in your palette, including neutrals in shiny solids or glittery weaves. Your prints are bold, wild, vivid, or ethnic in geometrics, paisleys, or stylised designs. For dressy occasions, you can wear satin, crepe, heavy brocade, or metallics – any theatrical or striking fabric or texture.

Because of your height, you can add emphasis at the waist or even below, such as dangling belts or lavish trim on a hemline. Your jewellery should be bold, simple, and large, or elaborate and ornate. Your hair, too, may be severely simple (short or long), ornately curled, or sleeked back in a chignon. Makeup applied theatrically works for you, for dramatics are not conservative types. On you almost anything goes.

Dramatics are usually Winters or dark Autumns. Most Summers and Springs who are tall and angular are best to go for a sophisticated rather than a dramatic look. It's just too severe for their softer colouring. Typical dramatics are, Diana Rigg, Diana Ross, Lauren Bacall, Barbra Streisand, Shirley Bassey and Liza Minnelli.

SPORTY/NATURAL

The sporty/natural woman is the casual type. Her build can range from tall and sturdy to tiny and boyish. Often she has wide-set eyes and a squarish jaw, or, at the other extreme, the face of a pixie. She may be athletic, but even if she's not, she has an energetic stride and an informal, friendly manner.

If you are a sporty/natural, you look good in all kinds of sportswear, from casual to chic. You can wear boots and leather, skirts and sweaters, tailored suits with top-stitching. Bouclé, natural, and hand-woven fabrics are good for you, as are tweeds, tartans, checks, and paisleys. Your prints should be large, casual designs. Solids are great for you, too, especially in textured fabrics. For formal occasions you are best in plain-coloured matt-finish fabric, such as heavy crêpe, raw silk, jersey, even quilted material.

If you are a mini-natural, the same rules for fabrics, checks, and prints

Sporty/Natural

Dramatic

apply, but you must scale everything down to your smaller size and wear lighter-weight fabrics. You have a youthful quality, and it is important for you to look perky and smart. For more formal wear you should choose 'young' fabrics like crisp, sheer cottons and velveteen. All natural types should avoid shiny fabrics or any theatrical look.

The sporty/natural woman is best in simple jewellery and not much of it. Makeup is minimal and natural and hair needs a casual cut and can look wind-blown. The tight, curly perm works well for some.

The Autumn palette lends itself especially well to the sporty look, though women of any season can be the sporty/natural type. Farrah Fawcett, Petula Clark, Candice Bergen, Carol Burnett, Goldie Hawn, and Virginia Wade are the sporty/natural type.

ROMANTIC

Romantic women should seek femininity in both style and fabric. The romantic woman has a curvy figure and looks best in clothes that have gently curved lines, with either a crisply full or a softly draped silhouette. Her fabrics should be luxurious and soft, with a sheen, and her prints should be rounded in feeling and design. Because she has striking colouring, the romantic woman may dress with theatrical flair, though she must take care not to look overdone or gaudy. She may wear exaggerated styles and sophisticated prints as long as they are feminine.

The romantic often has a beautiful face or a special facial feature, such as her eyes or complexion, and should choose necklines, accessories, and accent colours from her palette to draw the eye to her face. She looks beautiful in evening wear, and her rounded figure is shown to its best advantage in a low-cut neck-line and, if she's slim, a fitted waist. For evening, she is good in chiffon, silk, lace, shiny satin, brocade, velvet, and many other sophisticated fabrics, simple or ornate.

Jewellery for the romantic woman must be delicate in detail, though it may have a luxurious look. Her hair is best in curves or curls, even if she sweeps it off her face, and her makeup can be strong if it is not overdone. The romantic is often the woman who will take the time to put on false eyelashes.

If you are overweight, your best look may be romantic. Your extra layer adds roundness and softness to your body, so it would be unharmonious for you to wear clothing with severe lines. Curling your hair, wearing makeup, and wearing the colours from your palette that most flatter you will draw the eye of the onlooker away from those extra pounds and up to your face. Unless your body type says no, try this feminine approach to dressing. It has worked successfully for many of my clients.

Romantics come from all the seasons. Elizabeth Taylor is a Winter romantic; Ann-Margret, Autumn: Zsa Zsa Gabor and Marilyn Monroe, Springs; Peggy Lee and Judith Chalmers, Summer. The romantic look requires maturity, so if you are still in your twenties, dress for femininity, but save the theatrical for later.

INGENUE

The ingenue is the youthful romantic: pretty, dainty, delicate in build and colouring. The ingenue also needs feminine styles, curved lines, soft or crispy fabrics, and delicate prints. She looks good in floral prints, especially those that are animated or outlined. However, she is not theatrical or flamboyant, and her figure is youthful. She looks best in hair styles with curves or curls – soft, loose, or tight. She has a fresh, unsophisticated, natural femininity and should wear dainty jewellery and minimal makeup. She is best in her softer colours and lightweight fabrics with a matt finish. Sheer, crisp cotton, voile, organdie, broderie anglaise, thin jersey, or any youthful fabric is suitable for evening wear. Heavy, shiny, or glittery fabric is too overpowering for the ingenue.

The ingenue eventually matures out of this girlish look, usually becoming the more sophisticated romantic or a classic. She never becomes dramatic or sporty. Spring women are most likely to be the ingenue type, and, though a young feminine woman of any season may be an ingenue, Spring seems to stay that way the longest, probably because of her delicate colouring. Helen Hayes, Debbie Reynolds, and Jane Asher are all Springs who remained ingenues well into their 'prime'. The main point to remember, if you are this type, is that eventually you must give up ruffles and bows for a more mature look.

CLASSIC

If you have even, regular facial features, medium colouring, and a well-proportioned body, you are the classic type. The classic woman is tailored, conservative but smart, always well groomed. Typically, she has good posture, a sense of formality, and poise.

The classic woman avoids extremes in fashion, fabric, and prints. She is a scaled-down dramatic, avoiding trendy fashion and severe, straight lines, but achieving distinction through fine fabric, soft, straight lines, and immaculately tailored clothes. A full or crisp silhouette is not for her. The classic stays up-to-date in a conservative way: her hemlines go up and down just a little and she switches to the latest look only after it has become established.

Ingenue

Romantic

Fabric for the classic woman may be shiny or matt, but not too-heavy. Fine cottons and jerseys, fine wool and wool crêpe, fine knits, and brushed cotton (like Viyella) are all good. Prints, again, must be middle-of-the-road: small to medium, stylised designs, paisley and polka dots. For a Summer classic, a watercolour effect is nice. A Spring classic can have a more animated print, perhaps outlined to make it stand out from the fabric. Winter and Autumn classics look good in paisleys, stripes, conservative geometrics, or patterns that repeat evenly. For after six, the classic is good in chiffon, crêpe, silk or subtle brocade. A smooth or fine fabric is always better than one with a rough texture.

If you are the classic type, you must choose a controlled hair style that you can keep neat. The casual, windblown look is incompatible with your image. Your hair may be straight or curled, but not extreme. No Afro hairstyle for you unless you are black, because an Afro is classic for a black woman. Your makeup, too, must be conservative, but *do* wear makeup. The same is true for your jewellery. It should be of average size, subtle, but smart and chic. And *do* wear jewellery, especially earrings. Because the classic woman is 'medium' everything, she must be careful not to look plain, dowdy, or matronly. If you wear enough makeup, jewellery, and accessories to look smart, you can find the classic look exciting.

Classic

Although everyone can wear classic clothes, this look does not suit everyone equally. A woman with a dramatic face or body will look boring in classic clothes, while a voluptuous, romantic woman will look severe. However, we all become more classic as we age.

The late Princess Grace of Monaco, Vera Lynn, Margaret Thatcher, Princess Alexandra and Nancy Reagan are typical classic women.

ACHIEVING SEVERAL LOOKS

Many women can achieve several looks successfully. Sophia Loren can dress romantically or dramatically with equal credibility. Faye Dunaway can be natural or dramatic, and, with her hair in soft curls, romantic. Put her in a softly tailored suit and a short, controlled hair style, and she's classic.

Whatever look you favour, just be sure it is believable on you. When Jackie Kennedy Onassis was the President's wife, her image-makers tried to force her into a classic mould, in tailored suits, pillbox hats, and gloves. She looked constrained. The real Jackie, a sporty/natural, emerged in later pictures perched on the rail of a yacht with her hair blowing in the wind.

Of course, some occasions call for you to achieve a certain look – romantic, sporty, or conservative – in order to be dressed appropriately. Then you must adapt the required look to your style. You may be best in classic clothes, but when you're going to a rugby match you want to look sporty. While a track suit would not be right for you, a tweed jacket with solid-colour blouse and slacks would do the trick.

PRINTS

Your choice of prints and checks is very important in achieving your look. When selecting them, always scale the design to your size and height. A tall woman would normally wear a large print unless she has a very delicate bone structure, in which case she would be better in a medium-size print. A short woman with a sturdy build would also choose a medium-size print to blend her height with her body structure.

Often a print contains colours from more than one season. You can still buy it as long as you use the following guidelines:

1. The wrong colour should not dominate the print.
2. The wrong colour should not be too close to your face.
3. The print should not require you to wear accessories, such as shoes, from another palette.

Some women are not their happiest or best in any prints. There's nothing wrong with that. Stick to solids and use jewellery, belts, scarves, or interesting fabrics to add variety to your outfit.

DRESSING FOR BUSINESS

At the office, regardless of your type, classic is best. A business suit or a conservative dress is appropriate, especially while you are striving to establish yourself. Be sure your suit is in one of your colours, however. The popular grey suit theory is fine for Winters and Summers, but an Autumn or Spring in a charcoal grey suit will not create her best impression. You can achieve the same look in your own colours. Keep your makeup and jewellery modest. Be well groomed, but not flamboyant.

Even in a business environment, you can express your individuality to a degree as long as you do it conservatively. A dramatic woman can modify her suited look with a longer skirt, heavier jewellery, or a stronger print or colour in her blouse. A romantic woman can wear a softer fabric and a blouse of brushed cotton or silk/polyester rather than a crisp fabric. The sporty/natural can choose tweeds and a casual rather than silk shirt. Once you have proven yourself as a budding executive, you can take more liberties in expressing your clothing personality. But never dress too romantically at work unless you are aspiring for the boss rather than a promotion.

If you work in a field concerned with the arts, fashion, or women, you can wear less conservative clothing. You may in fact go further on the staff of a fashion magazine if you dress with more imaginative style and flair.

YOUR OWN BEST LOOK

Most of us draw from a blend of clothing types rather than choosing an extreme look of one kind or another. Rather than categorising yourself, observe yourself and see what really suits you.

Use the following list, marking all the looks you feel are for you. As you experiment, see which image gets you the most compliments. Check newspaper advertisements and clip out looks that you would like to try. One of my students taped these to her mirror to keep in mind the 'new person' she was becoming. She has become a veritable fashion plate.

Tick the looks that are best for you:

STYLES:	Me	Not Me	Try it
Severe, straight lines			
Soft, straight lines			
Soft, curved lines			
Full, crisp lines			
Billowy, blousy			
Clingy			
DETAIL:			
Contrasting: piping, buttons			
Crisp stand-up ruffles			
Soft ruffles, frills			
Pleats			
Soft pleats (folds)			
Bows			
Silk flower			
Lace			
Fur trim			

FABRIC TYPES:	Me	Not Me	Try it
Shiny			
Matt			
Smooth			
Rough			
Finely textured (weave or knitted)			
Bouclé (weave or knitted)			
Tweedy			
PRINTS:			
Large			
Medium			
Small			
Bold			
Moderate			
Subtle, blended			
Defined, crisp			
Sophisticated			
Casual			
From head to toe (dress, suit)			
From waist up or waist down (blouse, jacket, skirt)			

	Me	Not Me	Try it
JEWELLERY:			
Large			
Medium			
Small			
Delicate, simple			
Dainty, but lavish			
Abstract, modern			
Ornate, baroque			
Classic			
Hand-made			
HAIR:			
Severe			
Ornate			
Casual, windblown			
Soft curls			
Controlled curves			
Tight curls (perm)			
Straight			
High-fashion			
Conservative			

MAKEUP:	Me	Not Me	Try it
Minimal			
Moderate			
Elaborate			

Understanding your best clothing personality takes time, awareness, and trial and error. We are usually the last to see ourselves objectively, so be open-minded. Remember, too, to keep abreast of the changes you undergo over the years. You may be a sporty/natural at nineteen but a classic at thirty. Keep your image appropriate to your age. It isn't fun to dress too old when you're young, and it isn't flattering to dress too young when you're mature.

Explore the personality of clothing, and enjoy finding the look that is *yours*. With your colours and your most flattering image, you are on your way to being a totally beautiful woman.

CHAPTER SEVEN

FASHIONS, FIGURES AND FADS

Fashion is only as good as it looks on *you*. Some women seem to be able to wear the latest lines every year, but most of us cannot. The smart woman adapts the latest look to her own figure and personality rather than trying to alter her personal look to accommodate each trend.

Now let's turn to your figure and proportions and work on finding your best lines.

To start with, try not to become preoccupied with your flaws, but consider your assets instead. Don't be the woman who wears a jacket that comes down to her knees to cover a big bottom, or the one who refuses to smile and expose her crooked teeth. In the first case, you will look top-heavy and short-legged; in the second, you will look unhappy.

When you see yourself in the mirror, you probably zero in on blemishes, wrinkles, and bulges. All of them will seem to disappear when you learn to put together and project a total look that emphasises your natural colouring and your best features. The people you meet will see an attractive woman with a warm, genuine smile – not crooked teeth. Besides, perfect is boring.

The object of this chapter is to teach you to achieve that total look. You have learned how to make colour work for you. Now you will learn to select the lines and details that best complement *your* figure, proportions, and type.

Let's discuss the ways to deal with various figure problems.

POSTURE

Your posture dictates how good your clothes look on you; even the most expensive and beautifully fitted garment cannot overcome the unflattering effect of a slouching body. The lines of your clothes will hang gracefully if your shoulders are held erect and your tummy and bottom are tucked in.

Stand straight with your weight distributed evenly on both feet. Imagine a string running from your chest bone to the ceiling, suspending you like a marionette. Now drop your shoulders. Shake your head slightly from side to side. You should now be standing correctly.

Practise standing this way in front of a mirror, looking at yourself from the front and from the side. Practise walking while pulling up through your midriff, head carried high, shoulders down. When you walk, swing your leg from the joint at the hip rather than the knee. This stride is smooth and elegant.

PROPORTION

Understanding your proportions is the key to dressing yourself to your best advantage. Few of us have the perfect proportions that would allow us to wear almost anything, but we can create the illusion of average proportions by dressing in lines that fool the eye.

Ideally, your shoulders should be just an inch or so (2–3 cm) wider than your hips to allow the lines of your clothes to fall loosely over the hips from the shoulders. To determine your proportions, stand in stocking feet against a door and ask someone to make tiny pencil marks to indicate where each shoulder bone and hip bone is situated. Measure the distances between the marks. If your hips are more than an inch or 3 cm wider than your shoulders, or vice versa, you can take steps to give the illusion of a better proportion.

Next mark your height; then mark your leg length at the point where your thigh joint 'breaks' from the hip. Measure both distances from the floor. The average leg length is half of your entire height. If your measurements reveal a discrepancy of more than an inch or 3 cm either way, you will want to use some camouflage, though slightly long legs are often an advantage. Now, mark the door at your waist and your armpit. The well-positioned waist falls in the middle between your armpit and the leg 'break', and a variation of more than an inch or 3 cm defines you as either high-waisted or low-waisted.

Write down these measurements and keep your proportions in mind as we discuss the ways to flatter each part of your body.

Last, look at the size of your head in relation to your body. A small head gives the illusion of height, while a large head shortens. If your head seems too small or too large, adjust your hair style, making it either closer to your face to compensate for a large head or fuller for a small one.

FACIAL SHAPE

If the shape of your face is extreme in any way, avoid repeating this shape in your neckline. For example, a round face looks rounder in a rounded scoop neck; a square jaw is emphasised by a square neckline; and a long, thin face, especially one with a pointed chin, looks longer in a narrow V-neck. A contrasting neckline balances your face.

Minimises square jaw

Accentuates square jaw

NECK

If your neck is too long, very short hair will accentuate its length. For you, it's best to add some length, at least at the back, and avoid deep V necklines. You can wear scarves, mandarin collars, choker necklaces, or ribbons at the throat, and you are the lucky lady who can wear the generally unflattering cowl.

If your neck is short, an open collar, V, or scoop neck is your best. Avoid high or standup collars, polonecks, and cowls. A crew or small poloneck will work for you. Short hair is always your best bet, because it creates the illusion of distance between your head and shoulders.

Even with a short neck, you may wear scarves, but choose a soft fabric and a small size to avoid bulk.

Broadens wide neck   *Minimises wide neck*

To minimise a wide neck, keep a round or crew neckline close to the base of the neck on both sides. A gap on the sides adds width, which is fine for the average or thin neck, but not for you.

SHOULDERS

Shoulders come in three general types: square, average-tapered, and sloped.

Any neckline that is horizontal and shallow, such as a boat-neck, will make your shoulders look broader, and, if they are square, even more square. Conversely, the opposite line – deep and narrow, such as a V – will make shoulders appear narrower and less square. Avoid a halter top if you have either too-broad or too-narrow shoulders, as this line is unflattering to both.

If you have a shoulder problem, you can compensate by using these principles:

TOO BROAD OR SQUARE:

Wide and shallow neckline is unflattering

Deep neckline minimises

Narrow and deep minimises

TOO NARROW OR SLOPED:

Narrow and deep neckline is unflattering

Shallow neckline minimises

Wide and shallow draws the eyes out

A lapel is always more flattering than a plain neckline if your shoulders are not your best feature. Lapels that point up and out broaden the shoulder, while lapels that point down narrow them. Buy whichever kind is appropriate for you. Scale the size of your lapels to the size of your body. A large lapel on a tiny body is overwhelming, but a flouncy collar that extends over the shoulder bones is flattering to all shoulders and is appropriate even for the small woman if the fabric is not bulky.

Your shoulder seam is extremely important in creating the illusion of a good shoulder. A *set-in* sleeve is most flattering and can be adjusted to create a slimmer or wider look, depending on your need. For the broad or square shoulder, keep the placement of the shoulder seam right on the shoulder bone.

You may even cheat by moving the seam in a quarter inch (6 mm) if you have enough fullness in the sleeve to allow arm room. The overweight woman can look slimmer in clothes with a crisp, narrow shoulder line and judicious placement of the shoulder seam.

Your shoulder treatment affects the look of your entire silhouette. For the sloped or narrow shoulder, let the seam extend a bit beyond your shoulder bone, to widen. The seam will also give your shoulders the definition of shape they may lack. A woman with a very large bust also may use this trick to call attention away from her bust and draw the eye up and out.

Such sleeve styles as batwing, kimono, and raglan require a broad or squarish shoulder. The raglan, especially, tends to drop the shoulder downward, so women with sloping or narrow shoulders should avoid this line. It is even chancy on shoulders with an average taper, though you can alter the line of these styles by adding a lapel or collar that points up or out.

In sleeveless tops you should follow the same principle as with the shoulder seam. Keep the edge of the garment on the shoulder bone for broad or square shoulders, slightly beyond the bone for narrow or sloped. A sleeveless top with the line inside the bone will accentuate either problem. This line is best for the woman with good, average shoulders.

Any detail on a shoulder will broaden or accentuate it. Epaulettes, for example, should be removed from your outfit if you wish to minimise your shoulders, but they are great for adding dimension to shoulders that are too narrow, assuming an epaulette is your type.

Raglan   *Kimono*

Batwing   *Set-in*

There is no such thing as a right or wrong shoulder line, simply whatever is right or wrong for *you*! Remember, you are creating balance. Look in the mirror and ask, 'Do my shoulders balance my hips?' Perhaps the upward pointed lapel is okay because it is balanced by pockets on the hips or by a skirt with some fullness. The exception is the overweight woman, whose hips usually are wider than her shoulders and arms. She does best to create a 'slim' shoulder look rather than extending her shoulders to balance her hips. Later, after she loses weight, she can compensate for a too-narrow shoulder, if that becomes her problem.

Don't be afraid to be creative. Your dressmaker or your sewing machine has the power to improve the line of your outfit. Remove or add shoulder detail, change the direction of a collar, or change the placement of a shoulder seam. These are *not* difficult alterations, but do remember that you may need to lengthen a cuff if you're nipping in a shoulder.

ARMS

To determine whether your arm is long, average, or short, let your arm hang at your side, and look in the mirror. If your first knuckle aligns with your crotch, you have an average arm. Your elbow should be at your waist.

A wide cuff at the wrist shortens the look of your arm. If your arms are long, this is great; if they're short, avoid wide cuffs. A woman with long arms often has trouble finding sleeves that are long enough. Don't overlook the possibility of adding a cuff, even in a contrasting colour.

Everyone can wear a long sleeve, but the three-quarter sleeve looks best on a short woman or one with short arms. It is unflattering on long arms, on a woman with large hands, and on a tall woman who wants to minimise her height.

The short sleeve usually looks best if it falls one inch above or below the bustline, rather than right at the point of the bust. (If you are small-busted, it may not matter, however.) A sleeve ending just above the elbow can look matronly, especially if it has a rolled cuff or if your arms are heavy. In high-style clothing, this sleeve length can be attractive if you are slim and tall with average to long arms.

If your arms are heavy, avoid long sleeves that are tight or clingy – this accentuates fat.

BUST

Your bra can make or break the line of your outfit. Braless is fine for the woman with a youthful bust, but for the rest of us a bra is sexier and smoother. When you are wearing a bra, your nipple should be no more than three inches below your armpit (unless you are *very* full-busted). Take a good look at yourself to be sure your bra is doing its job. It may not be.

Many women make the mistake of buying the cup too small and the band too large. Get the snuggest fit around your rib cage that is comfortable, and the largest cup that still fits smoothly. In addition, women are built either far apart or close together, and bras are designed in both fashions. Be sure you are buying a style cut for you.

If your bust is very small, you will have to avoid necklines intended to show cleavage. But take heart. It is much easier to dress a small bust than a large one. You can wear high-style clothes and all the wonderful blousy designs that the large-busted woman must avoid. Be grateful for small blessings.

There is no escaping the fact that a large bust is a difficult figure problem, partly because it is hard to find clothes that fit. Here are some tips for the busty lady:

- Avoid sleeve lengths ending at the bust.

- Avoid horizontal lines at bust level – no seam, stripe, piping, or similar detail.

- Avoid a low yoke (or smocking) at the bustline.

- Try garments that taper gently under the bustline. Too much fullness adds bulk, and an outfit that is too fitted will accentuate your bust. Pass up a peasant blouse, which makes the figure fuller, in favour of a tailored blouse, which makes it slimmer. It is worthwhile to tailor or alter garments by adding a seam under the bustline, thus slimming the midriff, removing excess fullness, and adding the illusion of length between the waist and bust.

- Avoid high-waisted looks.

- Keep your belts small and, if possible, the same colour as your skirt or dress.

- Wear your collars open, and wear V necklines with lapels, rather than high necklines with no detail, such as polonecks or crew necks. Vertical lines – a necklace, a seam, a slit, small buttons – all help to minimise a large bustline.

WAIST

If you have a small waist, you're the lucky one who can have fun with belts. But if your tiny waist is in the middle of an hourglass figure – with large bust and hips – take care not to look too nipped-in or you will accentuate those other features. A gentle taper, with perhaps a tie belt, is your best look.

If your waist is wide, there's no point in calling attention to it. Use belts judiciously, keeping them narrow and the same colour or fabric as the garment. Or simply have a seam at the waist with no belt. Look for princess styles or high- or low-waisted dresses. Make use of the no-waist look with an overblouse or perhaps a second layer such as a loose waistcoat or sweater.

A short-waisted woman is also wise to use a narrow belt the same colour as the outfit or no belt at all. If your waist is high, you need to leave as much room as possible between your bust and your waistline. For you, a gentle taper under the bustline is effective in lengthening your midriff. When you wear separates, choose your belt to match your top, rather than your skirt or trousers. This trick adds length to your waist. Skirts and trousers cut without a waistband are your best bet.

For a long waist, do the opposite. Unless your waist is large, use wide belts that match the colour of your skirt, thus bringing the eye up. Choose skirts and trousers with waistbands, including high-waisted bands. You can also cheat a little with your waist seams, raising them a bit above your real waistline.

HIPS

Narrow hips allow you to wear high-style designs and any unisex jeans etc. But if your hips are considerably narrower than your shoulders, you need to strive for balance by adding dimension to your hips. You're the woman who can wear hip pockets or a full or gathered skirt. You are also one of the few who can wear a straight, box jacket, but you must balance this line with a pleated or flared skirt.

If your hips are too wide, avoid pockets or excessive fullness at the hipline. An A-line skirt works as long as it doesn't ride up, but an even better camouflage is a modified dirndl – not the lampshade you made in school sewing classes, but a very gentle gathering, about three inches (7.5 cm) more than the waistband, eased in evenly. Some slight fullness in skirt or dress is always good on you. But avoid cinching your waist. It's best to have fabric flow gently from waist to hips. Often a loose waistcoat or jerkin works well to camouflage a wide hip.

Long-waisted

Short-waisted

To flatter all hips, choose panties that give a smooth line to your garment. Bikini panties leave a ridge under slacks, unless you buy the kind with a wide lace band at the top. Smooth lines are youthful and sexy. The dent caused by bikini panties is not flattering. Bikinis are fine under loose garments. If you have trouble with a dent at the bottom of your panties, you may be buying them with leg bands that are too small.

If you need smoothing under slinky, revealing outfits, wear control-top tights or a very light weight panty girdle. A heavy girdle looks matronly and out-of-date and is not good for your circulation.

BOTTOM

An ample derrière limits the number of styles you can wear, but it is a fairly easy figure problem to cover. Choose skirts with some fullness or an A-line, rather than a straight skirt. Be sure your trousers fit properly, so they do not cup under the seat. The fit should be loose enough over your thighs to allow the fabric to flow smoothly from the bottom to the leg.

The style of your jacket is important, and a softly fitted jacket, moderately tapered, is always your best bet. A box jacket, with its straight lines, will not work with a large derrière, unless the jacket is short, above the crest of your bottom, and worn with a pleated or flared skirt. Avoid a box jacket altogether with trousers. A tightly fitted jacket is equally unflattering, because it accentuates the curve of your bottom. Never wear a too-long jacket in an attempt to 'cover up'. The length of your jacket must be determined *from the front;* it should be proportional to your total height and the length of your legs (see 'Legs' later in this chapter). A jacket that is too long for you only succeeds in making your legs look short and your body look top-heavy; you will ruin your total look. Instead, look proportioned and be sure your trousers fit properly at the back.

If your problem is a derrière that is too flat, you too need a skirt or dress with some fullness or a two-piece outfit that adds an extra layer of fabric where it counts. You may wear a tapered or box jacket, but a closely fitted jacket is too form-fitting. Why not let the taper of your jacket *suggest* what is (or isn't) really there?

If you have a flat derrière, one that droops, or a curved (sway) back, you will need to alter your trousers and skirts by removing excess fabric from the waistline at the back. A skirt that droops or cups at the back is unflattering to any problem bottom.

One final note on the bottom: by the time you are thirty, gravity has usually worked its will and your bottom has dropped quite a bit. Check your shorts and tennis dresses for length at the back as well as the front!

THIGHS

Heavy thighs are common, but they also are the easiest figure flaw to disguise. Skirts and dresses with an A-line or slight fullness provide easy camouflage, as do trousers that fit with ease over your thighs. Trousers that are too tight call attention to your thighs, revealing their shape and size, whereas a looser fit is slimming. Avoid trousers that taper at the ankle, as this silhouette emphasises the heavy thigh. The most flattering trousers line is a slight flare or a straight leg with a hint of taper at the knee.

If the current trend in trouser styles is not flattering to you, live out the season in skirts. Your best look will return another year.

LEGS

If your legs are short, avoid turn-ups on your trousers; wear high heels to give the illusion of length; and keep your suit jackets relatively short – no lower than the crotch, and preferably at the break of your leg. Your blouses and over-tops should be even shorter than your suit jackets for a balanced look. Remember, you are aiming for overall proportion.

High-waisted styles are excellent for the woman with short legs, as they give the illusion of longer legs and height.

Although slightly long legs are an asset, too-long legs make it difficult to find clothes that fit and to achieve a well-proportioned look. Do wear trousers with turn-ups and wear jackets that end slightly below the crotch when viewed from the front. Avoid high-waisted styles in trousers, skirts, and dresses (including wide belts). You are the woman who can successfully wear tunics, low-waisted styles (if your hips allow), and trim on your hemline.

If your legs are of average length, your best suit jacket length with trousers is at the crotch. In years when hem lengths are just below the knee, a suit jacket worn with a *skirt* needs to be shorter in order to look proportioned.

For most of us a three-piece suit, consisting of trousers, skirt, and jacket, is not a wise investment because the jacket will not be properly proportioned for both the trousers and the skirt. The exception is the tall woman, or the one with long legs, because her skirt is automatically longer and is thus proportioned to go with a longer jacket. But during years when hemlines are lower, a three-piece suit will work because the proportion of the skirt is increased.

Cuff minimises long legs

HEIGHT

The taller and slimmer you are, the more styles you can wear. The tall woman can wear heavier fabric, more fullness, and low-waisted styles, if her figure permits. If you are quite tall, however, 5'7" or more, you will do best to avoid all high-waisted lines, including short, waist-length jackets and vests. These lines increase the illusion of height and sometimes make the very tall woman look too tiny on top, again ruining the proportion of her total body. Use a full-length mirror to make the final judgment.

By contrast, the short woman looks especially good in high-waisted clothes and shorter-length jackets and waistcoats. A three-quarter sleeve, accessories or trim near the face, anything that draws the eye up, is good.

Attractive hem lengths are determined by your height as well as the shape of your leg. Midi-length hems shorten you and add weight, so wear longer skirts only if you really look attractive in them. A soft, floating fabric can be worn in a longer length than a heavy fabric. Looking in a full-length mirror, check the proportion of your hem to your size. Now look at your leg to see whether the hemline falls in a flattering place. (If you're wearing boots, you need only check proportion.) I use a piece of cardboard to determine flattering hem lengths on my clients. Hold the cardboard in front of yourself as you look in the mirror. Raise and lower it to see what happens to the shape of your leg. When you find a spot you like, have someone measure the distance from the floor. You can use this guideline for hemming all your skirts. Be sure you remember which shoes you are wearing, or, better yet, measure in stocking feet. Some women have slim, cylindrical calves and find that many lengths are flattering. But some of us have only one 'good' spot and are best to stick to it, allowing fashion trends to change us only slightly.

WEIGHT

The woman whose weight is normal can usually find lots of pretty clothes to suit her; she has to worry only about her special figure problems, if any. But if you are too thin or too heavy, you have a special need to create a *total* illusion, to enhance your overall look. In either case you should avoid clothes that are too tight and revealing; too-tight clothes accentuate both underweight and overweight bodies.

If you are extremely thin, you can soften the angles of your body and add dimension with some fullness in your sleeves and your basic silhouette, and by using prints and details. A simple tailored shirt on you is too plain, especially if you are tall. Give the eye more to look at by adding scallops to your collar, a large, special necklace or belt buckle, or perhaps interesting buttons or fabric texture. Just remember to scale prints, texture, bulk, and detail to your size; take care to be consistent with your clothing personality; and then have fun 'adding' to yourself.

If your problem is overweight, the most slimming trick is wearing your colours. A colour that flatters you draws the eye upward to your face and away from your body. Contrary to popular belief, black makes a body look larger. It is a heavy colour and silhouettes your body against almost any background – a light wall, for example. If you are a Winter, black is fine because it flatters your face and draws the eye up. It is true that large prints increase apparent body size, but a solid, bright colour – if it is *your* colour – can be slimming because it diverts attention from your body to your total look.

Tent dresses are the worst possible line for the heavy woman. These dresses usually have only two seams and excess fullness, neither of which is slimming. The more vertical seams your outfit has, the slimmer you look, and often it is possible to shed ten pounds with your sewing machine by adding 'fake' vertical seams. For example, I once bought a heavy denim skirt that stuck out like a tent and had only two side seams. The line was not flattering, so without removing the waistband, I stitched a seam up the front and another up the back, taking a few inches of fullness out of the hemline and tapering to just a thread at the

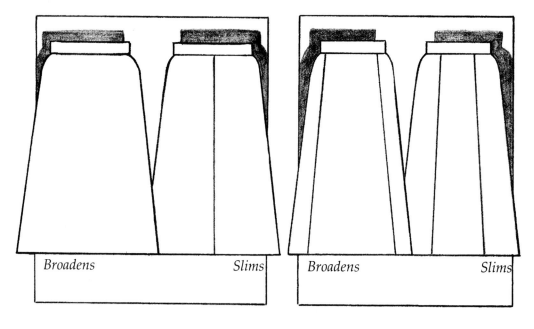

Broadens   *Slims*   *Broadens*   *Slims*

waistband. What a difference! We have done this in class for many clients, sometimes tapering a blouse, a skirt, or perhaps a whole dress.

When your outfit has seams, panels, or gores, keep them close together for a slimming effect. A wide-panelled gore in a skirt or dress creates the illusion of a wide body, while a narrow panel makes you look slimmer. (The too-thin woman can use these same tricks in reverse to add weight.)

In general, the overweight woman looks best in a line that is cut with ease but not excess fullness, and a fabric with a hard rather than a soft, clingy finish. Avoid bulky fabrics altogether.

If you dress carefully, people will see you as a whole, rather than zeroing in on your parts. Wear makeup, take care of your hair, and enjoy being pretty. There may be a diet and weight loss in your future, but meanwhile, dress to look your best right now.

CONCLUSION

Never worry about wearing the same line all the time, if that is the most flattering line for you. You can get variety through fabric, colour, and detail. No one notices the line of your outfit if it looks good, but people invariably notice clothes that are unflattering.

Again, remember that any fashion is only as good as it looks on *you*. If you follow fashion trends to be 'in', even when the current trend does not suit you, you are cheating yourself. But if you wear the latest fashion because it looks great on you, you've got the true fashion message.

And isn't it nice to know that while fashions and styles go in and out of vogue, you can go on looking your best year after year?

PART TWO

PUT IT ALL TOGETHER

CHAPTER EIGHT

YOUR FACE:
Finding the Right Makeup

You have established your colours, and you are ready to go. You've explored your clothing personality to see how best to express your individuality. Now it's time to put it all together, starting at the top.

The right colours on your face are every bit as important as the right colours in your clothing. One is incomplete without the other. You will never look your prettiest in makeup that is alien to your natural skin tone.

Many women who attend my classes have found shopping for makeup a source of frustration, and they often appear at the first class in the wrong colours. How well I remember the times I was sent home with peach foundation to 'match' my olive skin. What money I wasted on orange lipstick! Still ringing in my ears are the words of my aunt at that family reunion where I had wanted to look so good: 'You certainly do get pale living in the East, don't you?'

Now that you know your season, the mystery of makeup is solved and it is easy to know what makeup colours are right for you. Whether for foundation, rouge, or lipstick, the principle remains the same. The warm seasons wear peach, orange, and brick red; the cools wear pinks, plums, and true reds.

Makeup consultants are often trained to match your makeup to your clothes. Happily, you are now matching your clothes to you. By matching your makeup to you, also, you will find that one set – foundation, rouge, lip colour, eye makeup – will blend with everything in your wardrobe.

Even if you prefer not to wear makeup, don't skip this chapter. After working with women of all ages and tastes for years, I am convinced that every woman looks better and wears her range of colours more attractively with a touch of colour on her face. Some women need only a dash of blusher or a hint of lip gloss, while others need more. Colour, intelligently applied, maintains the glow of youth.

This chapter is primarily about colour rather than technique. If you are inexperienced at applying makeup, take advantage of the free advice offered at every major department store. The people there are experts at applying makeup; you will be the expert on what colour to apply. I have worked with many beauticians and, once they understand the palettes, they are delighted to learn about such a meaningful guideline to helping a client look her best.

As in all other aspects of fashion, beware of fads in makeup. Don't succumb to colours that don't look good on you. If brown tones are all the rage but on you look muddy, don't wear them. You can always be in style without sacrificing your best look.

SKIN CARE

Skin care is of course a must, and innumerable books have already been written on the subject. I will add only that in my years of study and consultations with dermatologists, both for myself and for my students, I have found two major fallacies in the method of skin care advocated by many cosmetics companies.

Fallacy No. 1: Everyone Should Wear Foundation. If you have clear, lovely skin that does not need smoothing, you do *not* need to wear a foundation. If you prefer no foundation, you can protect your skin by keeping it clean, sealing it with a toner, and moisturising it if necessary.

Fallacy No. 2: Everyone Needs Moisturiser. Not true. If you have oily skin or skin that tends to get spots, it is harmful to put any cream on your face. A woman whose skin consistently breaks out in spots should also avoid oil-base makeup – a water-base foundation is preferable. As you age, your skin will become drier, and eventually you will need moisturiser. Keep a watch on yourself, but don't be pushed into creams you don't need. Overmoisturising can actually cause your skin to sag.

FOUNDATION

Foundation, or makeup base, derives from two basic tones: rose (cool) and yellow (warm). Winters and summers wear foundations with a rose base, while Autumns and Springs wear those with a yellow base.

How do you tell the difference between a warm yellow beige and a cool rose beige? First, ask. Often the saleswoman knows her line well and is aware of yellow and rose bases. If she doesn't know, the name of the foundation can sometimes (though not always) be a clue. Yellow bases often are called 'natural', 'ivory', 'peach', 'golden', or 'copper', while rose bases are typically called 'rachel', 'rose', or 'sand'. Some names give no clue to the tone of foundation. 'Guadalupe Beige' is meaningless, so you will have to use your eye to judge.

Compare the beiges by putting a thick blob of each on your hand. A rose base will have a purplish or pink cast, whereas a yellow base will appear peach or yellow. You can see the tones when you are comparing shades. It's difficult to see tone in a colour standing all by itself unless the shade is extreme.

A Summer usually has noticeable pink in her skin and needs a base that looks pink and blends with her jawline. Some Winters also fall into this category, and these women rarely have difficulty finding a foundation. Many Winters, however, have either white, beige, or olive skin, devoid of visible pink tones on the face. These women need to be especially careful to find a beige foundation with a *rose undertone*. When a Winter erroneously finds herself in 'natural beige', she will look flat, perhaps a little sallow. If she ends up in peach, she will turn orange. Occasionally a Summer is sallow and needs to follow the same rule and avoid ending up in a yellow base.

If you are a Summer or Winter with a ruddy complexion, do not let a makeup consultant talk you into a yellow-base foundation in order to tone down your high colouring. Instead use a beige foundation that has no noticeable pink in it but that is derived from a rose base. This will tone down your ruddiness without detracting from your natural skin tone.

Depending on the depth of her colouring, the Autumn is best in ivory, peach, or copper tones. If she is just beige, she wears the 'natural beiges' with yellow undertones. A sallow Autumn does best with a peach foundation, if she is careful that it blends with her jawline.

A Spring most often wears a light to dark peach foundation. She should avoid blue-pinks. Some Springs are pure ivory and are best in an ivory base, adding peach to the cheeks with a blusher. Ruddy Autumns and Springs can tone down their high colouring with a warm 'natural' beige.

Some cosmetics lines are heavily weighted towards one base tone, and you may find nothing for you. Even the chemist who creates these colours is influenced by his or her own season, intuitively. Helena Rubinstein, before her death, was actively involved with the creation of her own line of cosmetics. She was a Winter. Now I know why I always had 'good luck' at her counter. So if you aren't finding what you need, don't hesitate to say 'none of these is right for me' and move on to the next counter.

Always check a foundation in natural light. Most stores have inadequate lighting, and what you see isn't what you get in the clear light of day. Test the shade of the foundation on your jawline. It should blend in perfectly when thinly applied. Never match foundation to your cheeks, as they have more colour than the rest of your face. Makeup matched to cheek colour will leave a line around the jaw.

Apply makeup thinly over clean skin that has been moisturised if necessary. Parched skin will absorb the foundation, giving you a heavily made-up look. Blemishes should be covered with a cover stick rather than a thick layer of makeup.

Do not spread makeup down your neck. Your neck is never the same colour as your face, and no one likes to see fingermarks of colour streaking down a lovely lady's neck. When blended perfectly to your jawline, the right colour will not show and will serve the purpose of smoothing the face.

Once you've found a good base, it will always be right for you and your clothing. With a summer tan, buy the same tone in a darker shade. Some women prefer to skip foundation in the summertime.

ROUGE

Rouge gives eternal youth, and it can be applied so naturally that only you and your mirror will know. Winters and Summers should wear rouges in the rose family, ranging from blue-pink to burgundy. Some Winters may prefer a clear red. Autumns need rouge in orange tones, preferably russet, ginger, or tawny peach. They should avoid pink-looking peach. Springs must stay delicate and wear clear peach, coral, or warm pink rouge, avoiding blue-pinks.

Creamy rouges are best for dry skin, and blush-on powders are best for oily skin. Gels are often difficult to apply, though the clear gel sticks are easy to manage and look extremely natural. They need to be reapplied periodically, as they tend to wear off.

Apply rouge or blusher along the cheekbone, beginning under the pupil of the eye and smoothing up into the hairline. Bring the colour down the hairline slightly and back to the original point under the eye, forming a triangle. Do not bring rouge lower than the bottom of your nose, in front, or into the circle area under the eye. Blend the edges for a natural look. Think of your face as a watercolour rather than an abstract painting. All colour should be applied sparingly and blended smoothly.

But if you lack cheek colour, be sure to use enough rouge; it is possible to underdo it. If you have high colouring, you can use rouge to reduce ruddiness, believe it or not. Nature seems to place cheek colour all in the front. It looks fine in the mirror because you see yourself only from the front, but others see you from the side. Add rouge to the sides of your cheeks to complete the triangle. You will be amazed at how this little trick distributes the colour, smoothing the cheek colour into your face.

Soften your rouge with age, as your skin lightens. Don't be a little old lady with two red dots on your face.

LIPSTICK

The same rules you used for foundation and rouge apply to lipstick or lip gloss colour: rose tones for the cool seasons, orange tones for the warm.

The intensity that is right for you depends on your age, the amount of colour you have in your lips, how dark or fair you are, and your clothing personality. Use the printed colour samples for your season as a guide when shopping for lipstick. Be sure to try out the lipstick testers on your lips rather than your hand, or you may be wasting your money. Very likely you will find one colour that is just right for you and will go with your entire palette. A lipstick does not have to match your clothes, as long as it blends.

Winter is the only season who usually needs to own two tubes of lipstick, one to wear with the true red of her palette and the other for the rest of her clothes.

Winter is best in pinks, plums, burgundies, blue-reds, and clear reds, avoiding orange or yellow tones. If your skin tends to make a lipstick turn blue, try a frosted lipstick, which often alleviates this problem. Remember that Winter in general needs clear, rather than muted, colours. Some Winters need a bright lipstick, while others can afford to wear a subdued shade. Although a few look attractive in brownish plums and burgundies, most do not. The exception is the black Winter, whose reds and burgundies do need some brown in them. But even these colours must have life to them for the Winter woman to look her best.

Summer needs a softer lipstick than her Winter counterpart. Her pinks, while blue, will be best in light shades. She may also wear burgundy and plum tones and, if necessary, cheat into a warm pink to avoid becoming too blue. The brownish pinks and plums are okay if they are not too dark.

Autumns should look for brick red, orange, coral, peach, rust, mocha, and brownish shades. Some Autumns need bright colours, while others need a soft, subdued colour. Autumns usually do not look good in highly frosted shades except for evening. They should avoid peaches that are too pink.

Spring may wear peach, warm pink, or coral. The pink should not be blue, and all of Spring's lipstick tones should be clear and not too dark.

Some Springs do well in clear red, though most are better in softer tones. Spring is not the brown lipstick type.

In the summertime, or any time you have a tan, select a lipstick a shade darker, but in the same tone as the one you normally wear.

When applying lipstick, it is essential that you master the use of a lipstick brush or lip pencil. It is difficult to follow your natural lip line accurately with a tube, even a new one. Just outline the lip line and then fill in the rest with the tube. If using a brush, buy sable; less expensive ones will soon have little hairs sticking out in all directions. Begin at the centre of your upper lip and follow the lip line to the left; then repeat from the centre to the right. Do the same for the bottom lip. Never stroke all the way from left to right in one swoop, or your lips will be crooked.

I do not recommend using a contrasting colour to outline lips unless you are striving for a theatrical rather than a natural look. If your lips already have a lot of colour, you can use a lip pencil to outline your lips lightly and then blend the line with your finger. The pencil outline, blended, also gives added definition to your lips if you wear lip gloss rather than lipstick. It takes a little practice to outline your natural lip line, but it's worth it. The use of a lipstick brush or pencil elevates your total look from 'almost' to 'arrived'.

EYE MAKEUP

Eyes are a beautiful, expressive part of a woman's face, and it is appropriate to accentuate their beauty. Yet many women make their worst errors in this effort. The object of eye shadow, for example, is to enhance the shape and colour of your eye. You want people to say, 'Look at the girl with the pretty blue eyes,' rather than, 'Look at the girl with the blue eye shadow!' *Never* let anyone tell you to make up your eyes to match your dress. That defeats the whole purpose of eye makeup.

EYEBROWS

Eyebrows should be plucked to follow the natural shape of the eye. Flat eyes usually are accompanied by flat eyebrows. Clean up the eyebrow area, but don't try to create a fake arch. Average to round eyes usually have arched eyebrows, and in that case plucking the arch area makes the brow attractive. Eyebrows growing toward the lid serve only to make the eye look smaller, so do pluck, but do it judiciously. Take a pencil and hold it against the outside of the nose and across the tear duct. The tip of the pencil will point to the place where your brow should begin. Now run the pencil from the nose to the crease at the outside of the eye to see

where the brow should end. Pluck out the excess or feather in the missing area with an eyebrow pencil. Do not pluck brows so that they become too thin.

If you need an eyebrow pencil, choose a colour based on your brow and hair colour. Try it out on your forehead. Winters and Summers need charcoal, brown, or blonde tones that have absolutely no red in them (even if the hair has red highlights). They should look for greyish or taupe tones. Autumns and Springs are the opposite and should look for golden blonde, reddish brown, or dark brown eyebrow pencils.

EYE SHADOWS

Eye shadows come in powders, creams, liquids, and crayons. Use whichever you personally find easiest to apply. I find powders the easiest to control, but they may accentuate crêpiness on dry or ageing skin. If you prefer crayons, be sure you use a creamy one that spreads easily. You don't want to stretch the skin around your eye area.

Eyes are of three general types: deep-set (with little or no lid showing), average (with some lid showing), and prominent or sunken (with most of the lid showing). Eye shadows can bring out or recess certain eye areas. A light shadow brings out an area; a dark shadow makes it recede. Each eye needs to be treated individually, but here are some basic guidelines.

For purposes of illustration, we will divide the eye into three areas from top to bottom: the underbrow, the orbital bone, and the lid. Some women need a highlighter shadow on the underbrow, a second shadow on the orbital bone, and a third on the lid. Others have eyes that have room for only two shades, a pale highlighter on the underbrow and a colour or darker neutral on the lid, brought slightly up onto the orbital bone.

Underbrow: A highlighter on the underbrow is a light neutral colour that serves to open the eye and clarify the skin, eliminating pink or tired brown tones around the eye area. Applying the highlighter from the brow to the lid gives you a good, clear base for the whole eye area.

Lid: On the lid, it's best to use a colour that blends with your own eye colour, but in a considerably softer shade. I do not recommend an eyelid colour that contrasts with your eyes. Having tested contrasting colours extensively, I find that they simply are not flattering and do not achieve the goal of making the eyes look their prettiest. Brown eyes are a slight exception. Brown eye shadow, while good on many brown-eyed Autumns and Springs, makes Winters and Summers look tired and drab. These brown-eyed types can use smoked mauve, plum, or navy to bring

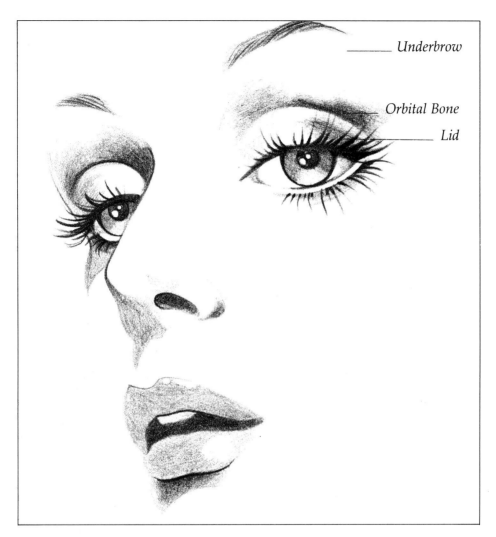

_____ *Underbrow*

_____ *Orbital Bone*
_____ *Lid*

out their eye colour – these provide a complement rather than a contrast.

A person with prominent or sunken eyes must stick to neutrals, rather than colours, on the lid. These might be brown, grey, smoked navy, or smoked plum, depending on the person's season and eye colour (see the charts that follow). Any colour-colour is glaring and calls attention to the lid rather than minimising it. For such eyes, apply the highlighter in the crease and the dark neutral on the lid just near the lashes, leaving the rest of the lid as is.

Orbital Bone: For most eyes, it's best to use a dark to medium neutral on the orbital bone. This neutral can also be brought down onto the outer third of the eyelid to widen the eyes a bit. A deep-set eye, with no lid showing when the eye is open, is the exception; it is sometimes effective to bring the eyelid colour onto the bone area, lightly. Just a hint of muted colour on the bone will bring out the colour of the eye. If it is too bright, mix it with a neutral.

Choose the eye type in the accompanying illustrations that most closely resembles your own and follow the principles when applying your eye shadow.

Now use the following charts to find the correct basic eye makeup colour for you. If your iris has two colours, you may use either. The lighter your skin, the lighter you apply everything. 'Dark', 'medium', and 'light' mean relative to you. Blend with a cottonwool ball or your fingertip. Remember, eye shadow means shadow, not bright colour. Even colour is used here to create a 'shadow' effect for a natural look.

If you wear glasses all the time, you may apply eye makeup a little more heavily than other people, but be careful not to overdo it.

Prominent

Average

Deep Set

WINTER Eyeshadow

Eye Colour	Brown	Brown-Green	Blue or Grey-Blue	Aqua-Blue	Green or Grey-Green
Underbrow (Highlighter)	Grey/Silver	Grey/Silver	Grey/Silver	Grey/Silver	Grey/Silver
Orbital Bone	Grey, Smoked Plum, or Smoked Navy	Grey	Grey, Smoked Navy	Grey	Grey
Lid	Mauve	Ash Green or Mauve	Ash Blue	Smoked Turquoise	Ash Green

If you are extremely fair, you may wish to substitute off-white for pale grey or silver highlighter under the brow. For the prominent eye, use smoked navy (which will appear grey when thinly applied) on the lid for brown and blue eyes, and grey or greyed green for green eyes. Above all, stick to cool colours with ash tones.

SUMMER Eyeshadow

Eye Colour	Blue or Grey-Blue	Aqua-Blue	Green	Brown
Underbrow (Highlighter)	Off-White	Off-White	Off-White	Off-White
Orbital Bone	Grey	Grey	Grey	Grey
Lid	Ash Blue	Smoked Turquoise	Ash Green	Mauve or Plum

Summers should not use dramatic eye makeup. Always blend well and keep subtle. For hazel eyes, pick the dominant colour and use that column. For green eyes, use a grey-green shadow even if your eye has some gold in it. Avoid yellow-greens, as you are striving for cool tones. Many blue eyes blend with a smoked turquoise better than with an ash blue shadow. You can tell easily by applying an excess of each colour, just to see which is better for you. Then blend. Occasionally a brown-eyed Summer will need smoked navy rather than mauve, plum tones on the lid, especially if her lid protrudes.

AUTUMN Eyeshadow

Eye Colour	Brown	Amber	Green	Blue (Turquoise)
Underbrow (Highlighter)	Beige or Apricot	Beige or Apricot	Beige	Beige
Orbital Bone	Brown or Copper	Brown	Brown or Muted Green	Brown or Smoked Turquoise
Lid	Brown or Beige	Brown or Apricot	Green	Smoked Turquoise

For hazel eyes, choose the dominant colour in your eye and use that column. For brown eyes, use golden or charcoal browns rather than red browns, which may make you look as if you've been crying. Beige is good on the deep-set lid. If you look tired in brown eye shadow, use a brownish green instead. Green-eyed Autumns should find the green swatch that most closely blends with your eye and find an eye shadow that is a softer version of that colour. Greens with yellow in them are best for you, but never select a bright green. Some Autumns can achieve a dramatic look in makeup quite successfully. But the more blonde and fair you are, the less makeup you should wear and the less dramatic should be your look.

SPRING Eyeshadow

Eye Colour	Brown	Amber	Blue	Aqua	Green
Underbrow (Highlighter)	Ivory	Ivory	Ivory	Ivory	Ivory
Orbital Bone	Golden Brown	Golden Brown or Apricot	Brown or Smoked Blue or Turquoise	Brown or Smoked Turquoise or Aqua	Brown
Lid	Brown	Brown or Apricot	Blue or Smoked Turquoise	Smoked Turquoise or Aqua	Green

Springs must apply eye shadow sparingly and blend it well. If you are extremely fair, rub most of it off with a cottonwool ball. Just a hint is enough for you. For hazel eyes, pick the dominant colour in your eye and apply the appropriate column. Your browns should be soft and golden – subtle, not dramatic. For aqua eyes, use a smoked turquoise or aqua rather than a bright one. Some blue-eyed Springs are better in turquoise than in blue. Green-eyed Springs look for yellow-greens rather than ash greens.

MASCARA:

Mascara is an excellent means of accentuating your lashes and toning down the eye shadow on your lid. It is best to use natural tones – blacks, browns, and blonde-browns rather than exotic colours. Again, you want to enhance your eye rather than call attention to your eyelashes. Apply mascara to your lower as well as upper lashes unless you have a protruding eye and wish to diminish its size.

Here are suggested mascara colours for each season:

Winter: Black (for extremely dark eyes only), brown-black, or brown, according to the depth of your colouring. Avoid red-browns.

Summer: Brown-black, charcoal, brown, taupe, blonde-brown, whichever is closest to the colour of your hair and eyebrows, but slightly darker. Avoid red tones.

Autumn: Brown-black, brown, light brown, whichever is best for you. Your mascara may have golden or red tones.

Spring: Brown, light brown, reddish brown, whichever blends best with your hair and brows.

EYELINER:

Eyeliner is not for everyone. Many eyes, especially deep-set or average types, look smaller when eyeliner is applied to the upper lid. But with the advent of smudgy pencils or crayons the line can be softened with your fingertip to serve as a deep eye shadow. It is effective on deep-set and average eyes to use a touch of crayon on the outer third of the upper lid.

The prominent eyelid needs eyeliner, in a neutral colour, smudged along the upper lid close to the lashes. This helps make the eye recede.

All eyeliners should be a neutral or smoky version of your eye colour – never a bright colour. The exception is liner for the eye that is so deep-set that the lid does not show at all. In this case you may use a crayon liner in the same colour as the lid eye shadow, applied thinly at the base of the lashes, then blended with your finger. This colour will barely show when the eye is open and will help bring out your eye colour. The woman with deep-set eyes, as I mentioned previously, can bring her lid colour lightly onto the orbital bone. Both of these techniques will 'open' her eye and enhance her eye colour.

All eyes except prominent ones can have the outer two-thirds of the lower lid underlined in a neutral colour: grey or charcoal for Winters and Summers, brown tones for Autumns and Springs. Keep it thin, blend it with your fingertip, and then apply mascara.

CONCLUSION

With a little experimenting, you will soon find just the right lipstick, rouge, eye makeup, and foundation for your colouring. All of it will fit in a little bag for easy portability. In fact, with so little makeup you can afford to buy two sets, one for home and one for your handbag.

These makeup guidelines are timeless. Whatever changes occur in the fashion world, you can retain your best look by adapting the fads or fashions to the colour scheme of your face.

Makeup is an important element in putting yourself together. It need not be expensive, and it should be easy and fun now that you have the confidence to know what's right for you.

CHAPTER NINE

YOUR HAIR:
Getting the Colour Right

HAIR COLOUR

One of the first questions women ask me is 'What colour should my hair be?' It's a good question, since many women who dye or highlight their hair are doing it in the wrong shade. In my classes I find that women want to colour their hair for one of three reasons: to stay blonde, to cover grey, to give themselves a boost.

Nature usually does it right, and for many, doing nothing is best. But sometimes it is appropriate to colour hair, and the secret to success is knowing what colour to select. Hair colour is simple once you know your season; any dye colour, or highlighting should go *with* your colouring, not against it.

Of all the seasons, Summers most often feel drab and want to enliven their looks by doing something to their hair. Often they were blonde as children, and their hair turned mousy as they entered early adulthood. I recall one especially beautiful Summer who had tow-coloured hair almost until her teens, and then it darkened. Instead of returning herself to her natural ash blonde colour, she succumbed to the latest fad at the time, red henna. Her hairdresser convinced her that it was the very latest and that this change would give her exactly the look she longed for. Henna on a Summer is harsh, ageing, and unharmonious with everything about her. It·clashes with her skin and her clothes. She must either wear the wrong makeup to go with the orange tone of her hair, or let her correct makeup clash with her hair. This beautiful Summer, who had not looked bad with her 'mousy' blonde hair, now looked terrible. All she had needed were her colours. A Summer's face comes to life when she wears her palette, and her hair will look livelier, too.

Summers and Winters, the cool seasons, should always strive for ash tones in their hair. Autumns and Springs, with their warm skin tones, will look best in golden or reddish tones.

WINTER

Most Winters have brown to black hair. Their hair is beautiful on them just the way it is. A Winter should *never* highlight her hair, nor should she bleach it blonde or add red. It can look striking if it is totally white, but achieving that look through the bottle is usually less than exciting because it looks artificial. Best to wait until it turns white all by itself. A Winter can use natural or black henna, but never red. If you are a Winter, do not let your hairdresser talk you into highlighting. Your hair is likely to turn red if stripped with peroxide, and the highlights will succeed only in making you look old.

The Winter woman's only question is what to do when she begins to grey. Winter is the season most likely to grey prematurely, and often the grey comes in attractively, creating a salt-and-pepper look. If you keep your hair short and chic, salt-and-pepper can be stunning. Long, unstylish grey hair is dumpy. If your personality does not thrive in grey hair, by all means colour it, but insist on ash brown tones when covering grey. Your hairdresser (or you) should not mix ash brown with any colour that has the word 'warm' in it. 'Warm' means that red will appear. Mix instead with ash blonde for a lighter, softer colour. A Winter can also use a grey shampoo or one of the shampoo formulas that cover grey naturally. A little grey left in the hair serves to keep it soft in tone. Remember that as you age, your skin fades and it is wise to let your hair lighten also. The rare blonde Winter usually stays blonde.

SUMMER

Summer's hair, whether blonde or brunette, often has a greyish cast that is beautiful with her Summer palette. The dark brunette Summer, like the Winter, should let her hair be. But a Summer who was once blonde or whose brown hair is light can be blonde successfully since she has a blonde complexion. Highlighting is an excellent way for the Summer woman to add life and blondeness to her hair. She should strive for ash tones, avoiding all flaxen, golden, honey, or red tones, including henna. The Summer often greys attractively and may wish to leave the grey for a naturally highlighted look. If she wishes to cover it, she must use ash blonde or brown tones and avoid all labels with the word 'warm'. A few Summers have a reddish cast to their hair due to the intense red pigments in their skin. (Summer men often have ash blond hair and red beards!) These Summers can use a grey shampoo to tone down the red if they wish or leave the highlights as they are.

Some Summers need contrast but want to be blonde. Ash blonde comes in many degrees, so don't forget the possibility of dark ash blonde for facial contrast, with pale ash highlights for 'glamour'.

AUTUMN

The Autumn woman is the one who looks terrific in red highlights. An Autumn who was a blonde child and wishes to stay blonde should always use golden blonde tones. Ash blonde will make her pale and will not harmonise with her face and clothes. For the other Autumns, auburn, red, and warm brown tones are the best shades. They should avoid ash tones. Redheaded Autumns should never let their grey show until they are completely grey. As grey hair comes in on an Autumn, it tends to be yellow-grey – ageing rather than chic. But once an Autumn's hair has turned completely grey, its overall warm tones can be most attractive. An Autumn is wisest to stay away from ash highlighting.

SPRING

Many Springs have warm blonde or brown hair that has darkened to a golden shade and looks beautiful just the way it is. If a blonde Spring wants to stay blonde, she should use flaxen or golden blonde hair colouring, never ash. A Spring is the youthful type and should not use any hair colour that looks too sophisticated or appears grey. Her hair does not grey attractively, and she is wise to colour it during its 'coming in' years. But once it is completely grey, or white, its warm colour is flattering. To cover grey, Spring can use auburn, golden brown, or golden blonde hair colouring. Some Springs are redheads and should keep that red hair forever. Look for the word 'warm' on a bottle of dye.

Appropriate Hair Colour			
WINTER	*SUMMER*	*AUTUMN*	*SPRING*
Ash Brown	Ash Blonde	Golden Blonde	Flaxen Blonde
Blue-Black	Ash Brown	Golden Brown	Golden Blonde
If grey,	Highlighting	Red-Brown	Golden Brown
her choice	If grey,	Red	Red-Brown
	her choice	Strawberry	Strawberry
		Cover grey,	Cover grey,
		unless hair	unless hair is
		is completely	completely
		grey	grey

HAIR STYLE

For hair style you should consider five points: your type, the shape of your face, the kind of hair you have, how handy you are with it, and your life style. A good hairdresser is your best friend, and you must give him or her as much information as possible about you and your hair. Discuss your facial shape and your life style. He or she is trained to help you achieve flattering lines. If your face is long and thin or rectangular, you will want to add fullness to the sides of your face. If it is round or square, you should minimise the sides. If you run into a stylist who wants to give you the 'latest' without regard to how it looks on you, find another one. Don't hesitate to insist that you are the classic rather than the dramatic type if you are being urged to have a frizzy and you feel it isn't for you.

An excellent cut is a must. I have moved many times over the last fifteen years and one of my first problems is finding a good haircut. My best tip, tried and true, is to keep an eye out for someone whose hair looks the way you would like yours to look and ask who her hairdresser is. Most people, even strangers, are flattered to be asked and are happy to share this information. But remember that some hairdressers are best at cutting certain types of hair – naturally curly, limp and straight, thin or

Thin Face   *Square/Round*

thick. For this reason it is best to find a woman whose hair is of similar texture to yours. Spend money on your haircut. A good cut makes all the difference in your daily appearance.

Long hair is fine for young women, but after thirty-five it is ageing. Then it is best to keep shoulder length the limit, or wear a style swept off the face. After all, gravity tends to pull the face down, so we need to keep our hair on the 'up' side. The older the woman, the shorter the hair. Many men love long hair, and I have had students in their middle years who keep long hair to please a husband or friend. Perhaps the reason is the youthful or sexual connotation of lengthy locks, but in both cases too-long hair defeats the purpose. Shorter hair on an older woman is both more youthful and sexier. Hair is a marvellous tool with which a woman can express her sexuality and how she feels about herself. Women who neglect their hair or wear an unflattering style are telling the world they are afraid to be beautiful.

You hair style can date you, so do keep abreast of fashion. If you are wearing the same hair style you wore ten years ago, you undoubtedly look less youthful than you could. By the same token, wearing an 'in', super-short, severe cut when you are a romantic needing femininity and curls is sacrificing your beauty to fashion. Be fashionable, be chic, but always be yourself. Adapt the current trend so that it works for you. The right hair colour and style work wonders for your total appearance.

CHAPTER TEN

A WARDROBE THAT WORKS

Having a wardrobe that works is easier than you think. Let your colours create it for you. With a plan and your palette you can have a coordinated wardrobe that will serve all your needs with fewer clothes, but more to wear. You will not have to ponder every purchase; you can rest assured that whatever you buy will blend with everything else in your wardrobe, thus saving you countless hours of shopping and countless pounds in 'mistakes'. The financial benefits of shopping from your palette are dramatic.

One client whom I had not seen for over a year telephoned to tell me how thrilled she was with the way her colours were working. 'I just bought one skirt, and I gave myself seven new outfits,' she said. The skirt was a print in a myriad of colours from her palette, and already in her wardrobe were seven tops in several of the colours, ranging from a casual poloneck to a dressy chiffon. The versatile cotton velveteen fabric of the skirt lent itself to dressing up or down. 'I was shopping for several parties and thought I would have to spend much more to fill so many needs,' she added. 'I already have the right shoes, evening bag, and jewellery, according to my wardrobe plan. I can't believe how well my wardrobe is falling into place.'

Because you undoubtedly already have some clothes in colours that are not from your palette, your wardrobe will not be completely coordinated overnight. But if you stick to your colours from now on, you will gradually produce this transformation. Phasing out wrong colours takes from two to five years, depending on what you currently own and how much you have to spend.

Make your old things work by mixing with a blouse, a scarf, or a waistcoat from your palette. Don't buy anything new from a palette that is not yours. The full benefit comes once your entire wardrobe consists of only your colours.

The *approach* to planning a wardrobe is the same for every woman, whether she is a busy mother or an executive, has a limited budget or money to burn, makes her own clothes, or lives in designer fashions:

1. Evaluate Your Life Style. Write down your usual routine over a normal two-week period. Add your evening activities and any hobbies or sports in which you participate. It takes only a few minutes to do this. Use your diary to refresh your memory.

2. Start with Basic Clothes and Keep It Simple. A good wardrobe revolves around a few essential clothes in your season's neutral or basic colours. It's easy to add extras according to your needs. I like to keep my wardrobe relatively small. As soon as clothes hangers slot in with difficulty, I know I've got clothes in the wardrobe I'm not wearing.

To begin, let's look at the work potential of your palette. Each palette contains colours for every occasion. You have neutral colours, basic colours, and accent colours, colours for the beach, the bedroom, and the boardroom; colours for day and colours for evening; colours for

	WINTER	*SUMMER*	*AUTUMN*	*SPRING*

Neutrals:	White
	Black
	Navy
	Grey
	Taupe
		Soft White
		Rose-Beige
		Rose-Brown
		Greyed Navy
		Blue-Grey
			Oyster White
			Beige
			Camel
			Dark Brown
			Gold
			Bronze
			Olive
				Ivory, Cream
				Clear Beige
				Camel, Tan
				Golden
				  Brown
				Clear Gold
				Warm Grey
				Light Clear
				  Navy

Basic Colours:	Burgundy
	Blue-Red
	True Red
	True Blue
	True Green
	Emerald
	  Green
	Pine Green
		Burgundy
		Raspberry
		Grey-Blue
		Deep Blue-
		  Green
		Blue-Red
		Watermelon
			Forest Green
			Moss Green
			Orange-Red
			Bittersweet
			  Red
			Rust
				Clear Red
				Orange-Red
				Coral
				Periwinkle
				Rust (some
				  Springs)

wintertime and colours for summertime. You plan your wardrobe, year round, from your palette, choosing a colour that is appropriate for that time of year.

Use the chart opposite as a planning guide:

Neutrals form the foundation of your wardrobe because they go with everything. Basic colours are the ones that are versatile and go with many others. Most are not too memorable and can be worn over and over again. Red, although bright, is a basic colour, since it mixes well with neutrals and many other colours.

Choose your most flattering neutral or basic colours for your coat, suit, jacket, and basic dress, the clothes worn closest to your face. Any of your neutrals may be used for skirts and trousers, shoes and bags. Generally, the darker neutrals are for wintertime, the lighter ones for summer.

The rest of your palette contains colours suitable for blouses, leisure wear, and accents. These are less versatile colours and are fine for extra dresses, skirts, or trousers, but they must be acquired *after* the basics.

SURVIVAL WARDROBE

Now let's discuss the most basic possible wardrobe. I call it a survival wardrobe. If you have one of each item listed, you have something to take you anywhere. Because this is a skeleton, it works for winter or summer clothes; simply adjust the fabric and sleeve lengths to suit hot or cold weather. We will add accessories to the plan later.

Your life style dictates how you expand or alter this basic wardrobe plan. The working woman should add another jacket, two additional skirts, several blouses, and one or two more versatile dresses, the kind that can go from day to evening with a change of accessories. The nonworking woman needs more trousers and casual clothes. If parties play a big role in your life, add more evening clothes in several neutral or basic colours before adding one in a bright colour. Some of my younger clients are students and say they have no need for evening wear and never wear dresses. Eliminate what you don't need, but be careful. One dress is a minimum for almost any woman's wardrobe. You might, after all, get an unexpected invitation from someone exciting, and shopping in a rush often results in a compromise.

If your figure lends itself better to dresses than skirts, or to skirts than trousers, simply substitute one for the other. A skirt and blouse ensemble often fills in for a dress. By the same token, a dress may be worn with a jacket to create the effect of a suit. Adjust according to your needs, keeping in mind that the first five items, plus a coat, are a must for any workable, ready-to-go wardrobe.

As you go through the list, put a tick by each item that you feel is necessary to your life style. Right now, don't think about what you *have*, but consider what you *need*. Write a zero by the items that are unnecessary for you, and a number by the other items, estimating how many you think you should have. If your life style varies considerably from winter to summer, make two columns. Later you will go through your wardrobe and see what you have and what is missing.

Last, add a section for special categories. If you are an avid golfer, tennis player, skier, or jogger, you will have special wardrobe needs.

Everyone needs a few old clothes for painting the garage or digging in the garden. Most of us already have these, but do make sure yours are in your colours. Why not be flattered in even your most casual attire!

BASIC SURVIVAL WARDROBE

_____	**Jacket**	Your first suit jacket or blazer should be in a neutral, solid colour from your palette with buttons to match. Keep the style simple for maximum versatility. Because this is the backbone of your wardrobe, the fabric and tailoring should be good. In the wintertime you might choose velvet, which is suitable for daytime or evening.
_____	**Skirt**	This skirt can be in the same colour as the jacket or a contrasting neutral. It is best to keep it solid, but a tweed will work.
_____	**Trousers**	The same rules apply to trousers. A solid is more versatile for the first pair and is dressier than a tweed. These should be in a good fabric, wool for winter, cotton or linen for summer.
_____	**Dress**	The first dress must be versatile, for daytime or evening. Keep the style simple, without a lot of trim or detail, and the colour solid, in one of the neutrals or basics of your season. Wool blends jerseys, cotton jerseys, and suede-look fabric are good choises for wintertime, while jerseys, silk, silk-like blends, and cotton knits are flexible for summer or warmer climates. Once the first basic dress is acquired, you can add prints and more memorable colours.

_____	**Blouse I**	A tailored blouse in a solid neutral or basic colour to go with your trousers, skirt, and jacket is the first on your list. The fabric should be of silk-like polyester, silk, or jersey – something not too casual but not too dressy for work.
_____	**Blouse II**	This blouse can be more casual, in a print, check, or solid accent colour, but in a less dressy fabric. It turns your jacket and trousers or skirt ensemble into a suit that could go to a football game or any sports event, while still being appropriate for work or casual occasions.
_____	**Dressy Blouse**	A blouse in a shimmering or sheer fabric with a bow at the neck or a blousy cut turns your skirt or trousers into a dressy outfit. This blouse should also be in a neutral or nonmemorable colour, and can be worn with evening trousers or a dressy evening skirt to stretch your wardrobe further.
_____	**Sweater**	A sweater in a basic colour adds another dimension to your wardrobe. It goes with your suit (with skirt or trousers), and as a separate with your basic skirt or trousers, and with your jeans and casual clothes. Try a poloneck or cowl (if a cowl suits you) for wintertime and a short-sleeved, cool knit for summertime.
_____	**Evening Trousers, Skirt, or Dress**	Evening trousers or skirts represent the most flexible approach to dressing up. Either should be in a basic colour and a dressy, versatile fabric, such as a 'silky' jersey, to go with your dressy blouse. You can add other tops, especially one in the same colour as the skirt or pants, for maximum dressiness. An evening or cocktail dress is fine, though it is not as versatile as separates. If you can have only one smart party dress, it must be in a neutral or basic colour. Your second purchase may be violet, fuchsia, or bright yellow-green. It will be remembered and cannot be worn as often.

Day to evening dress

_____	**Casual Trousers or Skirt**	This item can be of any casual material, from wool to denim, something comfortable that suits your life style. It can be more colourful, although, again, your *first* purchase should be relatively flexible. One outfit that falls in this category is trousers with a top or 'leisure jacket' to match. This combination is strictly casual and should not be confused with a trouser suit, which has a tailored jacket and can be dressed up to go almost anywhere.
_____	**Casual Shirt**	Add a T-shirt, cotton blouse, sweater, poloneck, or whatever you're comfortable in to go with your casual skirt or trousers. Most people need to extend this skeleton plan beyond one of each in the casual department.
_____	**'Old' clothes**	You need 'old' jeans, cords, shorts, T-shirts – whatever suits your fancy. Do toss out your wrong colours here, as clothes like this are inexpensive and some people's life style calls for jeans most of the time. Don't cheat yourself out of looking good on a daily basis.
_____	**Basic Coat**	In the wintertime, a basic coat for day to evening should be in a solid-colour wool, with matching buttons, in a classic, simple style. This coat is one of your major purchases, and you want it in a good quality and a style that is not quickly dated. A good, classic coat can last many years. Your basic survival wardrobe needs only this coat. You can add the following coats as your budget allows.
_____	**Casual Coat**	A casual coat is next on your list and can be a colourful wool, a trench coat, or even a leather coat. This coat should be fun, something to wear everyday. The working woman needs a trench coat, as it is businesslike, warm, and most useful in rainy climates. Others can wear a shiny oilskin in a bright colour to combat the rainy day.

A versatile wardrobe

_____	**Jacket**	Most of us also need some type of jacket, especially to wear with trousers. This could be a wool jacket or even an anorak, depending on where you live. If your money is tight, skip the jacket.
_____	**Evening**	Last, you will need something for evening. Your basic wool coat will do, but a velvet jacket or a fur (fake or real) would be your ultimate acquisition for a complete wardrobe. A fur is most flattering if it harmonises with your hair. Although brown is not in the Winter's palette, she can wear brown fur if she is brunette. Both Winter and Summer should take care to avoid red tones in any fur, and women of these two seasons look lovely in white fur as well. Autumns can wear the red and red-brown furs. Spring is great in creamy tones or in any golden brown or blonde fur. Use your swatches and your hair to guide your choice in fur. In the summertime, or in warm climates, a light trench coat or perhaps just a suit jacket in a light-coloured neutral will serve for daytime or casual evening, and for dressier occasions a pretty shawl is almost always appropriate.
_____	**Special**	Make a list here of your special clothing needs, the items you need for sports, hobbies, and so forth:

_____

_____

_____

_____

_____

_____

_____

_____

_____

_____

_____

_____

_____

_____

_____

_____

These items should fulfil your basic clothing needs. It isn't possible to anticipate every event, but as soon as you are able to have one of everything as a minimum, you will find that your wardrobe can handle most of the surprises that pop into your life.

On the following pages you will find suggested colours for your basic survival wardrobe. These suggestions are merely to show you how well your colours work together. Notice that your jacket goes with your trousers, skirt, and dress, and your blouses go with everything. Substitute other colours from your palette, according to your preference and their availability during any given year. As you build on this skeleton plan, add more colours. Even one new blouse adds a new dimension to your wardrobe.

It makes sense to acquire first the things you need the most. Later, you can add that slinky at-home outfit you saw in the lingerie department, or some fad item you're dying to acquire. In a year or two, after you have a start, you will be able to add more fun things to your wardrobe.

Try to buy ahead of need. When you shop, keep an eye out for the items missing from your wardrobe, even though you may not need them right this minute. Then, when you do receive an invitation or an opportunity, you won't have to rush out to shop.

Remember, the purpose of your colours, aside from making you look your best, is to simplify your life. So let your plan and your palette deliver their promise, and you'll have a wardrobe that really works.

WINTER SAMPLE COLOURS FOR BASIC SURVIVAL WARDROBE

	Wintertime	*Summertime*
Jacket	Black	White
Skirt	Grey	White
Trousers	Black	Navy
Dress	Red	True Green
Blouse I	Icy Grey	True Red
Blouse II	Purple, White, and Black Paisley	Navy and White Stripe
Dressy Blouse	White	Purple
Sweater	Magenta	Navy
Evening Trousers, Skirt, or Dress	Black	White
Casual Trousers or Skirt	Navy	White
Casual Top	Red	Shocking Pink
Coat	Black	(above jacket)
Trench Coat	Taupe (Grey-Beige)	Icy Grey
Evening Wrap	Emerald Green (velvet)	White (shawl)

SUMMER SAMPLE COLOURS FOR BASIC SURVIVAL WARDROBE

	Wintertime	*Summertime*
Jacket	Blue-Grey	Soft White
Skirt	Blue-Grey	Soft White
Trousers	Soft White	Greyed Navy
Dress	Raspberry	Sky Blue
Blouse I	Grey-Blue	Blue-Green
Blouse II	Plum, Navy, and Rose Print on Soft White Background	Red, White, and Navy Print
Dressy Blouse	Mauve	Pastel Pink
Sweater	Blue-Red	Light Lemon Yellow
Evening Trousers, Skirt, or Dress	Burgundy	Soft White
Casual Trousers or Skirt	Cocoa	Grey-Blue
Casual Top	Deep Blue-Green	Watermelon
Coat	Greyed Navy	(above jacket)
Trench Coat	Rose Beige	Powder Blue
Evening Wrap	Burgundy (velvet)	Soft White (shawl)

AUTUMN SAMPLE COLOURS FOR BASIC SURVIVAL WARDROBE

	Wintertime	*Summertime*
Jacket	Dark Chocolate Brown	Oyster White
Skirt	Coffee	Oyster White
Trousers	Camel	Beige
Dress	Rust	Lime Green
Blouse I	Beige	Yellow-Gold
Blouse II	Kingfisher Blue, Camel, and Chocolate Brown Print	Orange-Red, Turquoise, and Beige Stripe
Dressy Blouse	Beige	Salmon
Sweater	Bittersweet Red	Bright Yellow-Green
Evening Trousers, Skirt, or Dress	Dark Chocolate Brown	Beige
Casual Trousers or Skirt	Forest Green	Camel
Casual Top	Jade	Orange
Coat	Dark Chocolate Brown	(above jacket)
Trench Coat	Beige	Beige
Evening Wrap	Dark Chocolate Brown (velvet)	Beige (shawl)

SPRING SAMPLE COLOURS FOR BASIC SURVIVAL WARDROBE

	Wintertime	*Summertime*
Jacket	Ivory (or Soft White)	Light Warm Beige
Skirt	Ivory	Light Warm Beige
Trousers	Camel	Light Clear Navy
Dress	Red	Peach
Blouse I	Clear Salmon	Light Periwinkle Blue
Blouse II	Orange-red, Camel, Ivory Print	Bright Coral, Golden Yellow, and Navy in Tiny Floral Print
Dressy Blouse	Light Warm Beige	Warm Pastel Pink
Sweater	Golden Brown	Yellow-Green
Evening Trousers, Skirt, or Dress	Light Warm Beige	Ivory
Casual Trousers or Skirt	Golden Tan	Buff
Casual Top	Dark Periwinkle Blue	Light Clear Gold
Coat	Golden Brown	(above jacket)
Trench Coat	Light Warm Beige	Ivory
Evening Wrap	Ivory	Soft White (shawl)

CHAPTER ELEVEN

ACCENT ON ACCESSORIES

Accessories provide a fun and inexpensive way to create excitement in your wardrobe. If you have avoided them because you didn't think you knew how to choose them, your packet of colour swatches will now be your personal fashion consultant. You can hardly go wrong when buying shoes, bags, jewellery, scarves, or belts, because your palette is so compatible.

SHOES

Shoes should generally be in a neutral that blends with the colour of your skirt or trousers. A contrasting neutral is fine as long as the colour value is similar to or darker than the hemline of your skirt, dress, or pants. In the summertime or in a warm climate, you may break that rule with white or bone, depending on your season. Bright shoe colours must be repeated somewhere else on your body, preferably near your face. If you wear red shoes with a blue outfit, for example, wear a red scarf.

Build your shoe wardrobe on neutrals, then add the colours. In any given season you will find two or three neutral colours than will work with anything in your wardrobe. In wintertime, your choices might be as follows:

Winter	Summer	Autumn	Spring
Black	Navy	Dark Brown	Medium Brown
Navy	Grey	Tan	Tan
Burgundy	Rose-Brown	Olive	Navy

In summertime and warm climates, choose the following:

Winter	Summer	Autumn	Spring
White Black Bone (Taupe)	Off-White Bone (Rose) Navy	Bone (Yellow) Tan Brown	Off-White Tan Navy

Isn't it comforting to know that you *need* only two or three shoe colours? An Autumn has no need for navy; a Winter no need for brown. Of course, you may add shoes ad infinitum, if shoes are your thing; but most of us appreciate being free to spend our money on an extra outfit.

STOCKINGS

Four pairs of stockings or tights in a neutral skin colour keep you in stockings at all times. When one ladders, buy another. Buy your tights in the same colour. When one leg of them ladders, cut it off and save the top and the good leg. You can wear two pairs of one-legged tights at the same time, since the panties are thin enough to be comfortable when worn together! If you have two 'partials' of the same leg, turn one leg inside out.

The tone of your neutral stockings should be based on your season. Winters and Summers want grey-beiges or rose-beiges. Autumns and Springs wear golden beiges. Even your stockings reflect the totality of your look.

Dark or textured stockings or tights call attention to your legs and should never be worn if your legs are heavy. It is a fallacy that dark stockings are slimming! Only if you have very good-looking legs can you wear coloured stockings successfully. If you do wear them, use neutrals from your palette, of course.

BAGS

For everyday wear, you can have one basic handbag for wintertime and one for summer. The Winter does well with a dark grey bag, as it goes with black or navy shoes. Summer can use grey-navy; Autumn, medium brown; and Spring, tan.

Your bag should be in a neutral, either the same colour as your shoes or lighter. It does not have to match the shoe, but it must blend. Always draw the eye upward by having dark colours at the bottom (shoes) and lighter or brighter colours as you move up your body (bags, scarves). Moving upwards with accessories adds height, slims, and highlights your face.

In the summertime, Winters and Summers can use a white straw basket-weave, and Autumns and Springs a straw-coloured bag, which will go with everything and take you anywhere.

For evening at all times of the year, Winters and Summers should use a little silver envelope to go with all their cool colours, and the warm Autumns and Springs should carry a gold bag (you'll see why after you read about jewellery). Remember to keep your personality in mind when choosing bags and shoes. Both the size and the type should relate to you.

JEWELLERY

Here is your chance to make a personal statement. Your choice of jewellery reflects your type and your personality. We have already discussed the appropriate styles and shapes of your jewellery when we explored your clothing personality.

The metals in your jewellery are most important. White metals harmonise with the cool Winter and Summer colours, while gold tones harmonise with the warm colours of Autumn and Spring. You may be unhappy about that, but if you hold a piece of silver and gold jewellery against each of the palettes, you will see immediately which looks better. Notice how beautifully the silver tone blends with the Winter and Summer palettes? Now place gold against these palettes. You must admit, it clashes! Repeat the test by holding the gold against the Autumn and Spring colours: harmonious, luxurious, and right. Now the silver; it clashes.

The best jewellery for Winter is silver, platinum, and white gold; pearsls with a white or grey cast; white ivory; and white coral. And Winters look beautiful in diamonds! Summer uses the same white metals but may add rose gold, rose pearls (the expensive ones) and rose ivory. Autumns may wear any gold, brass, or copper tones, wooden jewellery, and tortoiseshell. They can wear the less expensive, cream-coloured pearls. Springs also need gold metals but must be careful to keep the colour and design delicate. Usually copper and brass are too bold for them. They are also best in creamy pearls.

You may wear any stones that blend with your colours. Use your swatches as a guide and set the stone in the metal of your season. The same is true for costume or enamelled jewellery. Your colours are a guide for everything!

Silver bracelets with gold trim

Pearls mix with
yellow or white gold

If you are young, you can begin collecting jewellery in the metals of your season, including your wedding ring! Many of us already have jewellery that's 'not ours'. however. As a Winter, I solve this problem by wearing my gold jewellery with the colours from my palette that are closest to the colours of the warm palettes: white, taupe, royal blue, and true red. You can do the same by wearing your 'off' jewellery with those of your colours that are close to colours from an 'opposite' season. It is possible to have your jeweller plate yellow gold with white gold and vice versa.

Yellow gold has a luxurious look that is hard to replace with a white metal; but mixing yellow gold with a white metal can give you the rich look you want without clashing with your palette. For example, you can mix metals in chains, bracelets, and two-colour earrings. For Summers and Winters, pearls are another answer. I wear pearl earrings as a basic, because they give a dressier and more elegant look than silver. Pearls can also mix with either white or gold metals. For a sportier look, silver is great. Autumns and Springs can achieve almost any look, from dressy to casual, with gold.

Buy earrings first, chains and necklaces second, a bracelet third, a ring fourth, and a brooch last. Start with earrings because they are what really make you look 'dressed'. In class, I keep some simple earrings on hand to demonstrate the effectiveness of this one accessory. A client is transformed from plain to chic with the snap of a metal clasp. Generally, an Autumn or Spring does well with a medium gold hoop or a button – smooth, brushed, or 'twisted'. A Winter or Summer can have a silver hoop, a button, or a large pear. Brushed metal is versatile because it can be sporty or dressy, while shiny metal is casual unless the style is quite elaborate.

Jewellery is best organised into groups. With a wardrobe of basics, you can use your jewellery and scarves to dress an outfit up or down. Plan three groupings of compatible jewellery: one casual, one dressier, and one formal. These can often be worn with the same dress. Simply change jewellery at five o'clock and you're set for an evening out. Here is a sample of groupings:

Casual (Shiny)	*Dressier* (Brushed)	*Formal* (Sparkly)
Shiny earrings in silver or gold	Brushed metal or pearl earrings	Earrings in pearls or a stone for your season
Informal brooch or casual necklace	Brushed metal brooch	Brooch or necklace with pearls or stone
Simple bracelet	Dressy bracelet or ring	Bracelet with stones; pearls; ring with stones

Be sure to add any missing jewellery items to your birthday or Christmas lists. Although it takes time to acquire jewellery, it is exciting to keep it in mind as something to look forward to. Husbands, friends, and family will appreciate knowing that their jewellery gifts are not only meaningful but also really suit you.

Try to keep any trim on your shoes or bags in the metal of your season. Often a shoe repair shop can replace one buckle with another. Sometimes, however, it isn't possible to find the right 'hardware', so choose a bag or shoe with minimal trim.

Always replace buttons with others of the right metal or colour for your season. That's easy.

SCARVES

Scarves are a vital part of your wardrobe; they are your means of bringing the right colour to your face while you are phasing the wrong colours out of your wardrobe.

Trims in metal of your season

Scarves are one of my favourite accessories. Even if you have a short neck, you can wear one, as long as you keep the fabric soft so it is not too bulky. A scarf can turn you into a fashion plate and add infinite variety to your wardrobe. A basic silk dress can go from morning to cocktails simply by clever scarf accessorising. Try a long, striped, multiculoured cotten (yes, cotton can mix with silk) sashed around your waist or twisted and knotted around your neck for a colourful, casual look, and switch to a soft, printed silk and dressier jewellery for evening.

A scarf can be draped in a thousand ways, and anything you invent goes if you wear it with confidence. Here are five effective ways to tie a scarf:

CLASSIC RECTANGLE

Fold a long, skinny scarf lengthwise until you have a band. Fold it in half, wrap it around your neck, and insert the ends through the loop formed by the fold. Pull taut and secure. Arrange at the front or off to the side.

ASCOT

Open a square scarf (large or small) and grasp the centre. Tie a knot right in the centre. Turn it inside out so that the knot is underneath. Take two opposite corners around your neck and tie at the back. Tuck the front into your collar and pin it to your bra.

Classic Square

Fan

Ascot

Twist

Classic Rectangle

FAN

Take a large square scarf and fold it back and forth until the entire scarf is pleated into one narrow strip. Holding the ends so the pleating won't fall apart, wrap the scarf around your neck and tie once in front. Do not knot, but secure with a safety pin or a stick pin. You have two fluffy fans, which may be centred or flared to both sides or off to one side. This is a spectacular feminine touch, a dynamite addition to any basic outfit.

THE TWIST

This technique requires a long rectangle and looks best if the scarf has a print, stripes, or multicolours, though it can be a bright solid. Knot both ends of the scarf near the edges. Twist and twist until the entire length of the scarf is a twisted rope. Keep it tightly twisted while wrapping it around your neck twice, bringing the ends to the front. Rather than tying them, tuck the ends into the rope, lapping them over and under until you have created an abstract 'knot'. This scarf trick is for the dramatic or tall, sporty type, and it does require a medium to long neck, but it's great fun if you can wear it.

CLASSIC SQUARE

Fold a square scarf on the bias and tie it with a knot around the neck, with the tails at the front or off to the side.

SECOND LAYER . . . AND A THIRD

Adding the extra interest of a waistcoat or jerkin or sweater is an inexpensive way to put zest into your whole look. Be sure to choose a fabric and style that suit your personality and figure. A loose jerkin can smooth the hipline and camouflage bulges. how about a waistcoat in a shimmery fabric to give your evening trousers or skirt yet another versatile twist? In wintertime, a long-sleeved sweater with a scoop or V neck over a solid or print blouse can really spruce up an otherwise plain skirt and blouse ensemble. Or try a blouse over a blouse, one tucked in, the other as a jacket. You can even add a third layer with a belt, tie, or sash if your figure permits.

HATS

Hats go in and out of fashion, and they're fun, if you are comfortable wearing them. Keep the colour lighter than or the same colour as your neckline.

When you try on a hat, stand in front of a full-length mirror; don't sit behind a table. Only then can you see its proportion in relation to your height and size. Don't forget to check the hat from the sides and back to see whether the shape is flattering.

A hat can increase or decrease the apparent size of your head if your head is small or large in relation to your body. Make these adjustments in the size of the brim, rather than the crown. The crown must fit your head accurately to look just right, but the brim may be any size as long as its not wider than your shoulders. A tall woman can wear a larger hat than a short one.

If you live where the winters are cold, pick a warm hat that goes with the coat or jacket you wear most of the time.

GLOVES

Since gloves are no longer mandatory for the 'well-groomed' look, you may not want to own any, other than a warm pair for winter. But if you do want a stand-by pair, your best choice is three-quarter-length kid gloves in the white or bone of your season. They can be crushed to wrist length and worn with any sleeve length.

Always keep gloves in a light neutral from your palette. Your hands move, and they are not the best place for a bright accent colour, except for outdoor sportswear.

Your warm winter gloves should be in a neutral to match or blend with your coat.

NAILS

If you wear coloured nail polish, your nails become an accessory, too. Colour calls attention to your hands, so stick to clear or buff if your hands or nails aren't your best asset. Otherwise, choose a nail colour that blends with your lipstick. It can be lighter or darker as long as it blends.

BELTS

A belt is a great way to add interest to an outfit. If you have a wispy waist, you can show it off with a wide belt or one of a contrasting colour. Otherwise, stick to narrow belts in neutral colours. A skinny belt in the metal of your season is a wonderful addition to your wardrobe. I consider it a basic, unless your waist says no. Even a large waist can have a belt buckle peeking out from beneath a waistcoat.

GLASSES

The frame of your glasses should be in the metal of your season, or in a colour that harmonises with your hair. As with fur colours, brown plastic frames are appropriate for a brunette Winter, even though brown is not in her palette. Again, Winters and Summers avoid red-brown tones.

The shape of your glasses should softly follow the shape of your face, but should not emphasise a pronounced facial contour. For example, if your jaw is square, your glasses should be squarish with rounded edges, rather than sharply squared. Proportion the size to your face, and keep the width of your glasses the same as your temples. Watch that your glasses do not go too far down your cheeks, or your face will look 'droopy'. It is best if the top of your frame is even with your eyebrows or a bit higher. If you can, take a friend when you shop for glasses, since it's pretty difficult to see yourself without the lenses.

If you want tinted lenses, choose a 5 or 10 percent tint the same colour as your eyes, unless you are a brown-eyed Winter or Summer. Like brown eye shadow, brown lenses may give these seasons a tired look. Brown-eyed Winters look great in mauve and brown-eyed Summers in rose, and these will look best with your clothes, too.

Sunglasses do not need to be as basic and can be in a metal, neutral, or any fun colour from your palette. If they are prescription sunglasses, you will probably want them in a neutral frame to go with all your summertime wardrobe.

CONCLUSION

Once you're dressed, stand back and take a good look in your full-length mirror. Do you need more, or less, or is your outfit just right? Accessories should be balanced, and no one accessory should be so bold that it detracts from your total look. Many women, however, are more likely to avoid accessories than to go overboard, for fear of looking overdone. Certainly, it's possible to go too far. One woman bedecked in too many brooches and bracelets is enough to scare anyone away from accessories permanently. Everyone knows the rule: 'When in doubt, don't.' However, this is your opportunity to be creative, so take a risk and *do*. But whatever you do, do it with confidence. Wearing accessories takes practice, trial and error. Have the courage to try a new look.

CHAPTER TWELVE

UNCLUTTERING YOUR WARDROBE

Now that you know what to look for, let's go through your wardrobe. Most of us are attached to our clothes, and it is hard to see them objectively. Ask yourself whether each garment in question still plays an active role. Allow time. You will never again have to spend this much energy on your clothes. From now on it will be much easier, so console yourself with that.

Four wardrobe problems crop up frequently.

Most common is simple accumulation of clothes, one outfit at a time, by the woman who buys for events as they occur. She has a shirt here, a pair of shoes there. Each was purchased to go with something now discarded, and it currently matches nothing. This wardrobe is a mix but not a match.

Then there is the wardrobe containing too many clothes. This woman buys impulsively, never gets rid of anything, and has decision confusion when it is time to get dressed or go shopping.

A third problem is common to the woman whose weight fluctuates. She has three sets of clothes, each in a different size, so she has both too many and too few clothes.

Last is the problem of too few clothes, either because the woman has financial limitations, or because she is depriving herself (feeling guilty or waiting to lose weight), or because she feels insecure about what to buy, or because her life style centres around blue jeans.

The first step in solving any clothes problem is to organise your wardrobe, so you can see what you have and what you need. The following guidelines will help you get uncluttered, as well as show you how to incorporate your season's colours into your existing selection of clothes, while phasing out 'wrong' colours as you can.

STEP 1

Remove everything hanging in your wardrobe that is not your current size. We are going to dress the body you have now. Even if you are left with three garments, that's all you have to wear anyway, so there is no point in making yourself miserable by staring at clothes that don't fit. Put the too-big or too-small clothes in another cupboard or in the attic, keeping only the ones that are still in style and are your colour. Stop waiting to buy clothes until you've lost weight. Look as good as you possibly can *right now.*

STEP 2

Remove everything in your wardrobe that you haven't worn for a year. I have consistently found that an item unworn for a whole year will not be worn this year either. The only exception might be an evening dress, because you haven't been invited to a formal party. Be ruthless. You are not doing yourself a favour having idle clothes taking up space. For each item, ask yourself: Is it your colour? Your type? A good style? If you haven't worn it lately, think of three good reasons for keeping it. Otherwise, give it to a charity shop or jumble sale where it can start doing someone else some good.

STEP 3

Separate your right colours from your wrong colours, setting aside the wrong ones for the moment. Organise all your right-colour clothing in groups, putting similar items together: jackets, skirts, trousers, tops, dresses, and so forth. If possible, line up your shoes and handbags so everything you possess is in sight. Now add the wrong-colour clothes that you feel are necessary to your wardrobe for now.

Any clothes in your wrong colours that you really don't love or need are best discarded. Often you can swap clothes with friends of other seasons. I gave my beautiful, expensive beige coat to a favourite Autumn friend, and when she weeded out her wardrobe she gave me a marvellous black leather handbag.

If you have too many clothes at this point, weed out excess duplicates. Twenty shirts are more than anyone needs. So are too many dresses, suits, or skirts, for that matter, regardless of how expensive or beautiful they are. It is of no advantage to either your wardrobe or your peace of mind to have an overwhelming number of clothes. I always suggest to the woman with too much that she create a skeleton wardrobe out of her favourite clothes, then add some extras and take a good, hard look at everything else.

STEP 4

Make yourself a chart to stick up in your wardrobe. I am including my favourite charts for you to hang there right now if you want, though you may need to make larger ones to give yourself more space for each category. One is for your wintertime clothes (page 145) and the other for summertime (page 146).

I also give a sample chart for a Winter's wintertime wardrobe (page 144) to give you an idea of how the chart should be filled out.

Fill in the chart that is appropriate for the current time of year, saving the other for later. Begin with the basics from your correct colours – jacket, skirt, trousers, dress. Then, in parentheses, add the clothes from your wrong colours, ones you feel are still good. The parentheses indicate to you that you will eventually want to replace these items.

The chart is designed so that you can mentally dress yourself. As you list your basic clothes in the left hand column, you can write in the appropriate shoes, handbag, scarf, or belt in the corresponding column at the right. Use a smaller version of this chart to plan your wardrobe for travel.

I like to number my shoes so I don't have to keep writing 'navy heels'. If some of your accessories are wrong for your season, keep only those that are essential during your transition period. Any stray shoes, bags, and especially scarves in the wrong colours should be given away. It is a blissful feeling to part with the last of the clothes that are not the true you. Then you are on the road to beautiful simplicity.

Underwear is included to remind you of special needs for those outfits that require a low-cut bra, a black slip, or whatever. I added that column after I had the experience of being on holiday with a brand new sheer dress and a waist slip that was far too short. I searched all over for a full-length white full slip and couldn't find one. I had to buy a camisole for the top and a floor-length waist slip that I cut off with some borrowed scissors. I thought about a slip the day I bought the dress, but I forgot about it while packing.

SAMPLE CHART

WINTERTIME WARDROBE

	Shoes	Bag	Scarves	Belts/ Hats	Underwear
Jackets BLACK (SUIT) NAVY BLAZER		(1) BLACK (2) NAVY		Burgundy HAT	
Skirts GREY WOOL BLACK WOOL (SUIT) NAVY GREY TWEED	(1) BLACK High (2) NAVY			BLACK BELT	
Trousers BLACK GREY TWEED	(3) BLACK LOW HEEL				
Blouses and Sweaters White, Magenta, NAVY, WHITE			BLUE; RED PAISLEY Burgundy PRINT		
Waistcoats/Slipovers NAVY					
Dresses BLUE ultrasuede BLACK Wool RED Wool	(2) (1) (1) or (2)	(2) (1) (1) or (2)			
Evening BLACK trousers, top ICE GREY DRESS PURPLE SILK DRESS	(4) Black, dress (5) Silver (4) or (5)	Silver bag '' ''			BLACK low cut bra Sandal foot Stockings
Casual: **Dresses** Burgundy velour Red Corduroy **Skirts** Denim Wool Check **Trousers** Jeans **Tops** Red Poloneck Green '' '' Black Sweater	(1) or (3) (3) (6) Navy (3) low heel (6)		Liberty print		
Coats BLACK WOOL TAUPE LEATHER FUR JACKET					

On the following pages are blank charts for you to fill out.

WINTERTIME WARDROBE					
	Shoes	*Bag*	*Scarves*	*Belts/ Hats*	*Underwear*
Jackets					
Skirts					
Trousers					
Blouses and Sweaters					
Waistcoats/Slipovers					
Dresses					
Evening					
Casual: Dresses Skirts Trousers Tops					
Coats					

SUMMERTIME WARDROBE

	Shoes	Bag	Scarves	Belts/ Hats	Underwear
Jackets					
Skirts					
Trousers					
Blouses and Sweaters					
Waistcoats/Slipovers					
Dresses					
Evening					
Casual: 　**Dresses** 　**Skirts** 　**Trousers** 　**Tops**					
Coats					

STEP 5

Make a list of the items missing from your wardrobe. After you see what's missing, arrange your list in order of priority, putting what you need most at the top. For example, you may find that while you don't have a perfect basic – a solid-colour, simple-style neutral – you may have something that will serve the purpose. Perhaps you have a houndstooth jacket instead of a solid, but it is giving you the suit you need for now.

This year a coat might be your priority. Because a coat is a major purchase, it may be the only thing you buy until next season except for a few accessories. Or you may feel you can wear your coat, even if it is the wrong colour, and put your money into a jacket or dress.

Your priority shopping list can be tucked into your handbag with your colours so it is handy when you go shopping. If you know you need a basic dress to complete your wardrobe, you can keep an eye out for it while shopping for other things. Don't forget to list the jewellery you want. Buying in advance of need is sensible rather than impulsive.

STEP 6

'Carry your wardrobe with you.' In our wardrobe classes at Colour Me Beautiful, the final accomplishment is 'having your wardrobe on a safety pin'! Here is the way we do it. Cut a three-by-five inch (7·5×12·5 cm) card into thirds. Then clip a bit of fabric from the seam allowance of each garment in your wardrobe and glue it to the card. If the fabric would unravel, write the colour on the card. Put your jackets on one card, trousers on one or two, then skirts, dresses, and so forth. Now assemble your cards on a safety pin, and you have your entire wardrobe to take shopping with you. Sometimes it's hard to remember what you've got at home, especially when deciding on tops or scarves. Your packet of colours takes the guesswork out of all your purchases.

With your wardrobe in order, you can begin to build sensibly. Updating a wardrobe from year to year is relatively simple. Perhaps you will add a slipover, a skinny overbelt, and a blouson dress or blouse to bring your last year's clothes up-to-date. Often it takes only an accessory, a silk flower, or one item in a 'new' fabric to keep you in style.

An uncluttered wardrobe and an overview of your clothing needs give you direction for shopping and for spending your money wisely. At the same time, with a little yearly weeding and updating, you will have a well-coordinated, easy-to-care-for wardrobe forever.

CHAPTER THIRTEEN

SHOPPING SANELY

Before I had my colours, I spent five years trying to buy a wool trouser suit. After living in California all my life, I was suddenly confronted with winters in cold New York, and trouser suits were coming into vogue at the time. The first autumn, I tried on everything in my size, but nothing seemed to look good and, after all, a good trouser suit is expensive. The next autumn I tried again, traipsing from shop to shop; and so it went, year after year. Finally I had my colours, but now I also had a three-year-old in nursery school. Any young mother knows that nursery school gives you two hours in which to accomplish all shopping, the alternative being shopping with a tired child. Armed with my packet of colours, I entered the sportswear department of my favourite store and in twenty minutes had picked out everything available in my size and colours – a total of five outfits. Only five, because it was autumn and the racks were full of the usual autumn colours. The third try-on was it – stunning – though the jacket needed minor alteration for a perfect fit. What a change! The culmination of a five-year hunt had taken just an hour and a half. I spent money on that purchase, but I knew it was right and wore the suit for years.

To shop with my colours as a guide is a pleasure. No wonder I had never found satisfactory clothing for myself in the autumn. Never realising that colour was the factor, I had blamed it all on style and fit, the bulkiness of autumn fabric, the terrible 'new' designs, the weight I had gained. Autumn is no longer intimidating. Now that I accept the fact that most years the autumn clothes will not feature my Winter colours, my eye looks only at what's for me and there is always something nice.

Here are some shopping 'Do's' and Don'ts' to help you save time and make your shopping decisions easy and rewarding.

Do: Shop with your colours, and look only at items in your colours.

Be sure you understand your colours. Familiarise yourself thoroughly with your palette and the colour concept of your season.

Always shop with your swatches. The eye cannot retain a colour image for more than a few seconds. It is difficult to tell whether that hot pink dress hanging on the rack is Spring's, Summer's, or Winter's, unless you have another pink for comparison. Put your swatch right up against the garment and, if necessary, take both to a doorway for better light. Often shop lighting distorts colour. Remember, you have some colour territories in which you can shop freely, using your swatches as a guide. But a few colours in each season must be matched as closely as possible if you are to look your best.

You will find that your own season will usually be the best time of year for shopping, as that is when your colours are most often presented. During the other three seasons, you will have less from which to choose, but as your eye becomes accustomed to spotting your colours, you will find enough. One terrific outfit in your colour is far more valuable than two in the wrong colours.

Occasionally, a fashion trend will be in your favour, enhancing your colour selection during your 'off' seasons. But some years will be better than others, so it is vital for you to build your basic wardrobe to carry you over a lean year. When designers are pushing muted shades, Winters and Springs will have to ferret out the few clear colours available. And that's the year for Autumns and Summers to stock up. When clear and bright is fashionable, Winters and Springs can buy for the future.

Long-sleeved blouses in year-round fabrics can be bought off season. I rarely wear long sleeves in the summertime because I live in a hot, sticky climate; but whenever I see a long-sleeved blouse in a colour that would be suitable for my wardrobe, I buy it. It may not be available in the autumn when I need it, because autumn usually means earth tones.

Autumns and Summers have the easiest shopping all year round; Winters and Springs must do more hunting. It's a small price to pay when the reward is guaranteed compliments and guaranteed good feelings about yourself. Besides, you will find that shopping is much faster now. Even if there is nothing for you, you will spend only a few minutes scanning the racks. You still have your money, your time, and your energy to check out another department.

You can take advantage of sales, knowing that whatever you buy at the end of this year's season will go with the unknowns you will buy next year. But remember your colours. A sale item is a bargain only if it looks good on you. A £2 scarf is a £2 waste if it doesn't flatter.

Do: Be aware of the fashion industry's colour cycles. Be open-minded about which of your colours you will buy.

Shopping with a specific colour in mind may lead to frustration and disappointment. The fashion industry pushes specific colours each season, and these, along with certain standard colours, are virtually the only colours available. If you are determined to buy a navy blue coat in a year when brown, grey, and burgundy are the fashion colours, you will only disappoint yourself. First see which colours in your palette are popular this year. Then choose the most flattering.

Understanding the fashion industry and its cycles is a great help in achieving your best look year after year. Buy your colours when you see them. Choose a classic style that will last and *build* a wardrobe.

Even though it is sometimes frustrating to cope with planned obsolescence and unpredictable hemlines, change is exciting, and we can appreciate the creative talent of designers who devote their time and energy to our clothes. And by pushing only a few colours each season, manufacturers can coordinate accessories – shoes, bags, jewellery – to complement the year's fashions. Imagine how confusing it would be if every colour were available all the time. The shops would burst their seams, and you would have a nervous breakdown sorting through the merchandise. Industry must offer selective colours, and it's a favour to the shopper, too.

We who know our colours do not have to worry about planned obsolescence. This year's shoes will go with next year's clothes because all our colours go with each other. Build that wardrobe and you stay in control, no matter what the fashion world is offering.

Do: Learn to say 'no'.

When you walk into a store, you are bombarded with merchandise, all saying 'Buy me'. By buying only colours from your palette, you impose a pleasant discipline on yourself. Rejoice in knowing what *not* to look at.

People can't hoodwink you into buying unflattering clothes unless you let them. When a salesperson says, 'That is the very latest; everyone is wearing it,' resist. You are not everyone – you are you. Buy fashion only if it really looks good on you. You can always be in style in your own special way.

Remember you have a perfect right to shop and try on as many garments as you like. The sales personnel are being paid to help you. They are already receiving compensation, so you do not owe them a purchase. How many of us have succumbed to sales pressure, buying something and returning it later when a different salesperson was on duty? I did. But no more. Your colours can give you the confidence to say yes or *no*.

Do: Find a salesperson who is your season.

People automatically like their own colours – salespeople included. Unless they are trained in colour, they will invariably show you the clothes that look good on them. Even when I hand a salesperson a packet of colours for myself or a client, I find that unless she is the same season, she will inevitably waste our time showing us innumerable wrong colours. Even though you show her your green, she will bring you clothes in her green. Find a salesperson who is your season, and she will become your shopping ally. She's the one who can run around finding you that red blouse because she knows where all the merchandise is hidden. Make use of salespeople. Most really do enjoy helping you.

Men tend to use sales personnel more than women. They are always in a hurry to get in and out of a store and are often happy to have a salesperson 'show' them what to buy to ease the decision-making process. It is essential for a man to have a salesperson of his season. On one shopping expedition, an Autumn salesman was helping my husband and me (my husband is a Summer). We asked to see blue suits, and the salesman kept showing us brown suits. My husband tired after five minutes – his usual shopping time-span – and began muttering 'let's go' while moving towards the exit. Hanging on to his shirt-tail so he couldn't escape, I was scanning the racks myself, knowing we had not seen all the merchandise. Our discouraged salesman wandered off, and along came another salesman, a Summer who whipped out a number of grey and blue suits, one of which we bought five minutes later. My husband's agonies are over, as his favourite Summer salesman does well for him every time.

I have been hired by department stores to train their salespeople, and the experience has proved that their new awareness of colour does make them more valuable to customers. Many stores, however, have not yet trained their salespeople to be colour sensitive. So, until that happy day arrives, choose your helper by colouring rather than by personality.

Buyers also dramatically influence the selections in any given store, so pay attention to the merchandise you generally see in the store as a whole. It may or may not be for you, depending on the season of the buyer. My Autumn friend finds everything she needs at a particular boutique where I consistently find nothing. Once I met the owner, who is also the buyer, I saw why. An Autumn, of course.

Don't: Shop with a friend unless she (or he) understands your season.

Shopping with a friend can sometimes be a hindrance to your best look because, unless she has her colours too and understands that you and she may be different seasons, she, like the salesperson, will intuitively steer you into styles and colours that are suitable for her, not you. Your colours are your best guides when you shop.

If you want the fun of shopping with a friend, be sure she understands your new colours. Spend some time discussing both of your types and personalities. Give her the test in Chapter 4 so she'll have her colours, too. Then you'll really be able to help each other.

Your favourite man has colour prejudices too, so be careful. He may love brown tweed and urge you to buy it without being completely aware of its suitability for *you*. If you're a Winter, and he wants you in tweed, show him you care in salt-and-pepper tweed or houndstooth – the look he likes, but the colour that's right for you. He'll be convinced the moment he sees how great you look.

Don't: Buy impulsively.

When shopping, work toward completing your basic wardrobe. Buy first the clothes you need most, using your priority list as a guide. If you see a dress you like, but you already have enough dresses, don't buy. Many of us accumulate the clothes we find easiest to buy for ourselves and consequently never reserve enough in our budget to buy something else we really need. If you have trouble finding trousers that fit, and you need trousers, resist that extra dress and keep hunting. On the other hand, when you see an item that is missing from your wardrobe, grab it, if your budget allows. This purchase is not impulsive. It's part of your plan.

Do: Spend the most money on the clothes you wear the most.

Invest your money in the clothes that really count. If you wear a suit only occasionally, it's fine to buy a less expensive suit and put your money somewhere else. But if you wear a suit to work every day, you need quality. It would be a mistake to squander your budget on an expensive cocktail dress for one occasion, if it means skimping on a suit. The suit must be of a good cut and fabric to hold its shape wearing after wearing. A lesser-quality garment in this case would be a poor investment, costing you more money in the long run because it would have to be replaced so quickly. Invest in the suit and hunt around for a less expensive evening outfit. You won't regret it.

Do: Be well groomed when you shop.

Dressing well when you shop gives you two advantages. You will be better able to judge clothes on yourself, and you will receive better service. It isn't fair, but it is true that salespeople will respond to you according to the way you look. If you wear dungarees and your gardening shirt when you shop for a nice dress, the salespeople will assume that you are a person with limited taste and/or no money to spend and they will concentrate on the woman who looks as if she will buy. Dressed carefully, I have often walked away with only a scarf, but much attention and solicitation from a fawning salesperson. Another time, dressed in jeans and a T-shirt, I have practically had to force someone to take my money for a rather expensive purchase.

You can best judge how a garment looks on you if you are wearing the right underwear, stockings, and shoes. If you are shopping for jeans, wear trousers; but if you are looking for a dress, suit, or evening gown, dress accordingly. It is impossible to decide whether an elegant evening dress is flattering if you're wearing socks and flatties.

Do: Develop a shopping routine.

Shopping by colour is the biggest timesaver in the world! It is a boon for the working woman or anyone who requires a complete wardrobe but whose life style leaves little time for shopping. First find your size. Then select the items in your colour. Third, check out the personality of each outfit – is it your type? Next, look at the style and cut of the garment. Now, feel the fabric; scrunch it to see if it wrinkles. Is it appropriate for the intended occasion and for your needs? Check the cleaning instructions. Labels give instruction on care, and it is disappointing to discover at home that the 'wash-and-wear' skirt you bought has to be dry-cleaned. Now try on the garment and check for fit. Don't overlook the possibility of alterations. Although colour works magic, a poor fit is still noticeable and detracts from your best look.

Get to know which manufacturers (or designers if you are lucky) consistently produce clothes that are cut well for you. With practice, you will be able to buy some clothes without even trying them on.

Shopping can be fun even if you don't have much time for it. Colour makes it easier, faster, and much more rewarding.

CHAPTER FOURTEEN

LET YOURSELF GLOW

Now that colour has changed your outer image, use it to change your self-image as well.

We have all seen the woman who, despite attractive features, perfect make-up, and immaculate grooming, radiates nothing. She looks good on the outside, but on the inside she feels like nobody, and that is the image she projects to others.

As you wear your colours, you can turn the good looks and the compliments into good feelings, so that you not only look your best, but feel beautiful as a person – and that's the ultimate winning combination. The special magic of colour is that your new image is authentically you, based not on fakery or 'beauty tricks' but on flattery of the real you. You are not hiding what you don't like about yourself; you are revealing the best of yourself.

Let's summarise the steps you take to find your natural beauty and put your colours to work for you.

1. Take the colour test to determine your season.

2. Study and understand your colours. 'Shop' with your swatches and get to know your colour 'personality'.

3. Start wearing your colours, beginning with what you have.

4. Start wearing the right makeup colours. Be particular about the shades. Correct makeup does make a difference and you need only one set.

5. Attend to your hair, in both colour and style. Get rid of the wrong colour as soon as possible. It really detracts.

6. Check out your wardrobe and list the things you need, keeping the list with your swatches. Buy new clothes in your colours only. Always shop with your swatches. Your eye cannot retain colour by memory and there are subtle differences in some shades.

7. As you shop, give thought to your type and the styles and accessories that most suit you. Watch for compliments as the signal you are on the right track.

8. Begin to build a wardrobe around basics.

Now, let yourself glow. The real fun comes as you develop your own sense of style, the look that says, 'I am me'. Style is not fashion. Style is the positive expression of your individuality, of both your inner and your outer personality.

Your colours alone do not give you style, but they help. It takes time and effort on your part to implement your new look and explore your clothing personality. But even if you don't develop a flair for dressing, you will achieve a statement of style and a put-together look from the dynamics of your palette alone.

As you wear your colours, you will find that you grow into your season and people begin to associate your colours with you, even in the gifts they choose for you. And you can use your colours to develop a style that can be expressed in every aspect of your life. Your home or office decor, the flowers you choose, your stationery, linens, china, even your wallet, umbrella, and car become a reflection of your own style and personality.

In your home, you can use your swatches to plan a colour scheme. If you live with someone whose season is different from yours, mix the two by putting together compatible colours from both. Usually it's best to stick to two colours in a room decor and then tie them together with a neutral or pale version of one of the two colours. For example, you might mix Winter's yellow with Spring's light orange on a rug of neutral ivory or pale yellow. Because yellow and orange are warm, use Spring's warm palette to add a print or a small touch of an accent colour. Your palette is an invaluable aid to decorating your home. It's rewarding – and flattering – to live in your colours, and be in harmony with your environment.

Develop your own ideas as you explore other ways to express your personality through your season. Here are some suggestions.

The Winter woman might choose flowers that are bold or formal – perhaps carnations or long-stemmed roses in colours from her palette. Summer's flowers would be softer – roses, gardenias, violets. Autumn might choose chrysanthemums, zinnias, poppies, and large daisies, while Spring's flowers could be daisies, daffodils, tulips, lilies of the valley, or baby rosebuds. Both the colour and the 'feeling' of the flowers in your home can reflect your personality.

Stationery for the cool Winter woman should be sophisticated, with perhaps a modern silver monogram. For Summer, the classic, traditional type with a script monogram is best. Autumn would choose rough paper with a heavy gold monogram, whereas Spring is most likely to be herself in delicate paper with a small, crisp monogram in gold.

Even your perfume personality can emerge from your season. While Winter is good in exotic, spicy scents, Summer is more the floral type. Autumn is best in woody or fruity fragrances and Spring in light, fresh, sweet smells from flowers or fruits.

Do you see how your palette can permeate your entire life style and even help you develop your identity?

So you are really not at the end of a book, but rather at the beginning of a whole new look, perhaps a new life. Colour is not static. It is vital and dynamic. The real rewards are still in your future. You can colour yourself beautiful in the truest sense of the word, with the glow – the beauty – that comes from total harmony and satisfaction with yourself.

INDEX